Workbook

Rau's Respiratory Pharmacology

T0091989

Eleventh Edition

Douglas S. Gardenhire, EdD, RRT, RRT-NPS, FAARC
Chair and Clinical Associate Professor
Department of Respiratory Therapy
Lewis School of Nursing and Health Professions
Georgia State University
Atlanta, Georgia

Sandra T. Hinski, PhD, RRT-NPS
Dean, Career and Technical Education
Academic Affairs
Paradise Valley Community College
Phoenix, Arizona

ELSEVIER

Elsevier
3251 Riverport Lane
St. Louis, Missouri 63043

WORKBOOK FOR RAU'S RESPIRATORY CARE PHARMACOLOGY,
ELEVENTH EDITION

ISBN: 978-0-323-87160-0

Notice

Practitioners and researchers must always rely on their own experience and knowledge in evaluating and using any information, methods, compounds or experiments described herein. Because of rapid advances in the medical sciences, in particular, independent verification of diagnoses and drug dosages should be made. To the fullest extent of the law, no responsibility is assumed by Elsevier, authors, editors or contributors for any injury and/or damage to persons or property as a matter of products liability, negligence or otherwise, or from any use or operation of any methods, products, instructions, or ideas contained in the material herein.

Previous editions copyrighted 2020, 2016, 2012, 2008, and 2002.

Content Strategist: Melissa J. Rawe
Senior Content Development Manager: Meghan B. Andress
Content Development Specialist: Kayla Jarman
Publishing Services Manager: Deepthi Unni
Project Manager: Sheik Mohideen K
Design Direction: Gopalakrishnan Venkatraman

Printed in India

Working together
to grow libraries in
developing countries

www.elsevier.com • www.bookaid.org

Last digit is the print number: 9 8 7 6 5 4 3 2 1

Contents

The Answer Key is included with text purchase and available at http://evolve.elsevier.com/Gardenhire/Rau/respiratory/

1 Introduction to Respiratory Care Pharmacology

CHAPTER OUTLINE

Pharmacology and the Study of Drugs
Naming Drugs
Sources of Drugs
Sources of Drugs
Process of Drug Approval in the United States
The Prescription
Respiratory Care Pharmacology: An Overview
National Board For Respiratory Care (NBRC) Testing Questions
Case Study

CHAPTER OBJECTIVES

After answering the following questions, the reader should be able to:

1. Define pharmacology
2. Define drugs
3. Describe how drugs are named
4. List the various sources of drug information
5. List the various sources used to manufacture drugs
6. Describe the process for drug approval in the United States
7. Define orphan drugs
8. Differentiate between prescription drugs and over-the-counter (OTC) drugs
9. Apply the various abbreviations and symbols used in prescribing drugs
10. Describe the therapeutic purpose of each of the major aerosolized drug groups
11. Identify related drug groups in respiratory care

PHARMACOLOGY AND THE STUDY OF DRUGS

Complete the following questions by writing the answer in the space provided.

1. Application of pharmacology to the treatment of pulmonary disorders and, more broadly, critical care is called a

   _____.

2. The study of drugs (chemicals), including their origin, properties, and interactions with living organisms, is called

   _____.

3. The time course and disposition of a drug in the body, based on its absorption, distribution, metabolism, and elimi-

   nation, is called _____ _____ _____.

4. The mechanism of drug action by which a drug molecule causes its effect in the body is called _____.

5. The study of toxic substances and their pharmacologic actions, including antidotes and poison control, is called

   _____.

6. The name assigned to a chemical, when it appears that the chemical has therapeutic use and the manufacturer wishes to market the drug, is _____ _____.

7. A virus that causes the formation of syncytial masses in cells and may cause respiratory distress in young infants is called _____ _____ _____.

8. _____ _____ is an organism that causes *Pneumocystis* pneumonia in humans and is seen in immunosuppressed individuals, such as those infected with the human immunodeficiency virus (HIV).

9. The art of treating disease with drugs is called _____.

10. A _____ is the written order for a drug, along with any specific instructions for compounding, dispensing, and taking the drug.

NAMING DRUGS

Complete the following by writing the answer in the space provided.

11. A _____ name is given to an experimental chemical that shows potential as a drug.

12. The _____ name indicates the drug's chemical structure.

13. The _____ name is what the generic name becomes once it receives official approval.

14. The _____ name is the nonproprietary name (*example:* Motrin; Tylenol).

15. Fill in the following different names for the antiasthmatic drug zafirlukast.

    a. Chemical name _____

    b. Code name _____

    c. Official name _____

    d. Generic name _____

    e. Trade (or brand) name _____

SOURCES OF DRUGS

Complete the following questions by writing the answer in the space provided.

16. What is an official source of information about drug standards if you want to obtain information about medications, dietary supplements, and medical devices? The U.S. Food and Drug Administration (FDA) considers this book the official standard for drugs marketed in the United States.

_____.

17. This reference source has lots of color charts that identify drugs, lists manufacturers, and tells how the drugs work, when they are indicated and contraindicated, and possible side effects.

_____

18. What subscription service provides monthly information on drug products and new releases?

_____

SOURCES OF DRUGS

Complete the following question by writing the answer in the space provided.

19. Most of today's drugs come from chemical synthesis. List three other sources that contribute to the synthesis of drug preparations with an example of each.

    a:_____

    b:_____

    c:_____

PROCESS OF DRUG APPROVAL IN THE UNITED STATES

Complete the following questions by writing the correct term in the blank provided.

20. Provide a brief description of each of the phases involved in the investigational new drug (IND) approval process.

    a. Phase 1:_____

    b. Phase 2:_____

    c. Phase 3:_____

21. After a successful IND process, a New Drug Application (NDA) is filed with the FDA, and a detailed reporting system is in place for _____ months to track any problems that arise with the drug's use.

Match each of the following definitions with the correct classification of therapeutic potential by placing the letter of the best answer in the space provided.

22. _____Important (significant) therapeutic gain over other drugs.

23. _____Modest therapeutic gain.

24. _____Important therapeutic gain, indicated for a patient with AIDS; fast-track.

25. _____Little or no therapeutic gain.

A = Important (significant) therapeutic gain over other drugs.

AA = Important therapeutic gain, indicated for a patient with AIDS; fast-track.

B = Modest therapeutic gain.

C = Important options; little or no therapeutic gain.

After each question, provide the correct answer.

26. Define the term *orphan drugs.*

27. When referring to orphan drugs, what does the term *rare* mean?

28. An orphan drug that respiratory clinicians use for the treatment of persistent pulmonary hypertension of newborns is called _____ _____ _____ .

29. Tobramycin, or TOBI, is an orphan drug used to treat in patients with _____ or bronchiectasis.

30. An orphan drug used to prevent or treat respiratory distress syndrome in newborn infants is _____ .

THE PRESCRIPTION

The prescription is the written order for a drug. It contains instructions for the pharmacist and patient about how to make, dispense, and take the drug.

Answer the following questions about the prescription.

31. Name the six parts of a prescription.

    a. _____

    b. _____

    c. _____

    d. _____

    e. _____

    f. _____

32. Give an example of an over-the-counter (OTC) drug.

33. Use Table 1.3 in the textbook to match the following list of abbreviations with their meanings.

    a. qd   _____   A drop
                                                 A spray
    b. bi   _____   And
                                                 As needed
    c. et   _____   By mouth
                                                 Cubic centimeter
    d. cc   _____   Every
                                                 Every day
    e. gtt   _____   Every hour
                                                 Every other day
    f. IM   _____   Four times daily
                                                 Intramuscular
    g. L   _____   Intravenous
                                                 Liter
    h. mL   _____   Milliliter
                                                 Nothing by mouth
    i. PO   _____   Three times daily
                                                 Twice daily
    j. q   _____

    k. prn   _____

    l. nebul _____

m. NPO _____

n. qh _____

o. qod _____

p. qid _____

q. tid _____

r. IV _____

RESPIRATORY CARE PHARMACOLOGY: AN OVERVIEW

Using Table 1.4 in the textbook, provide the answers for questions 35 and 36.

Complete the following question by writing the correct terms in the blanks provided.

34. List five advantages of aerosolized agents given by inhalation.

a. _____

b. _____

c. _____

d. _____

e. _____

Answer the questions by writing the answer in the space provided.

35. Drugs used to treat infections, such as antibiotics and antifungal drugs.

36. Agents paralyze people and are used in critical care.

37. Drugs used to help reduce the effect of pain by affecting the central nervous system.

38. Drugs that treat dangerous cardiac.

39. Drugs used to treat high blood pressure and chest pain.

40. Agents help keep blood from clotting.

41. Drugs used to rid the body of excess body fluid.

1. On reading a patient's medical history, it is learned the patient has a diagnosis of HIV infection. This would indicate the causative organism of the patient's pneumonia is likely
   a. *Pseudomonas aeruginosa*
   b. *Streptococcus aureus*
   c. *Haemophilus influenzae*
   d. *Pneumocystis carinii (jiroveci)*

2. Studies involving human subjects occur during which stage of the drug approval process?
   a. Chemical identification
   b. IND approval
   c. NDA
   d. Internal review

3. Which of the following is the generic name for the antiasthmatic drug Accolate?
   a. Proventil
   b. Zafirlukast
   c. ICI 204,219
   d. ED-AA

4. If you are looking up a drug in a reference source that has color charts that identify drugs, lists manufacturers, and tells how the drugs work, you are looking in the
   a. *Hospital Formulary*
   b. *Hospital Reference Source*
   c. *Physicians' Desk Reference*
   d. *Drug Handbook*

5. Which of the following is an advantage of aerosolized agents by inhalation?
   a. Aerosol doses are larger than those used for the same purpose and given systemically.
   b. Aerosolized agents have more side effects than those given systemically.
   c. Aerosolized agents have a slower onset of action.
   d. Drug delivery is targeted to the respiratory system and is painless.

6. An order has been written for a patient to receive an aerosolized bronchodilator tid. This would indicate the patient should receive the treatment
   a. Four times a day
   b. Three times a day
   c. Once a day
   d. Every 3 hours

7. An agent that will relax bronchial smooth muscle and reduce airway resistance to improve ventilatory flow rate in chronic obstructive pulmonary disease (COPD) and asthma is
   a. Adrenergic
   b. Corticosteroid
   c. Antiinfective
   d. Mucoactive

8. A patient has been ordered to receive a corticosteroid. This could indicate the patient has a need for
   a. Bronchial smooth muscle relaxation
   b. Thinning of mucus
   c. Increase in lung compliance
   d. Reduction and control of inflammatory response in the airway

9. This is an agent that is used to rid the body of excess fluid that may accumulate in the lungs.
   a. Antiinfective
   b. Antithrombolytic
   c. Diuretic
   d. Anticoagulant

10. As you enter a patient's room, you notice a sign above the bed that reads "NPO." This would indicate
    a. Administer medications by mouth only
    b. Administer drugs by IV only
    c. Nothing by mouth
    d. No needlesticks

11. This legislation put more controls on biologic agents and toxins and was passed in 2002.
    a. Prescription Drug User Act
    b. Supplemental Drug and Enforcement Act
    c. Bioterrorism Act
    d. Amendment Act

12. A class of drugs including montelukast and zileuton is used to
    a. Reduce infection
    b. Prevent the onset of asthmatic response
    c. Help increase surface tension in the alveoli
    d. Reduce pulmonary hypertension

13. A specific aerosolized agent used to inhibit or eradicate specific infective agents in patients with CF is
    a. Pentamidine
    b. Tobramycin
    c. Ribavirin
    d. Zanamivir

14. A prostacyclin analog used to treat pulmonary hypertension would include
    a. Iloprost
    b. Zileuton
    c. Lucinactant
    d. Beractant

CASE STUDY

An 8-year-old patient with CF has been admitted to the hospital. According to the patient's mother, this is his first hospital admission as a result of his CF. His CF has caused increased shortness of breath and more difficulty coughing up secretions. The following order has been written for respiratory care treatment:

Arterial blood gas stat

Albuterol 0.5 mL dil in 3.0 mL normal saline q4h and prn, et chest physical therapy p̄ nebul treatment qid

NPO 1h a chest physical therapy

Oxygen 2 L/min c̄ nasal cannula

1. Interpret this order, and identify the symbols and abbreviations used in this order.

2. During administration of the treatment, the mother of the patient asks why her son is receiving albuterol, because he has never used this medication. Explain.

   Change albuterol and normal saline treatment.

   After 3 days of respiratory treatments, the patient has improved, and a new respiratory order has been written:

3. What is wrong with this order?

2 Principles of Drug Action

CHAPTER OBJECTIVES

After answering the following questions, the reader should be able to:

1. Define key terms that pertain to principles of drug action
2. Define *drug administration phase*
3. Describe the various routes of administration available
4. Define *pharmacokinetic phase*
5. Discuss the key factors in the pharmacokinetic phase (e.g., absorption, distribution, metabolism, and elimination)
6. Describe the first-pass effect
7. Differentiate between systemic and inhaled drugs in relation to the pharmacokinetic phase
8. Explain the lung availability/total systemic availability (L/T) ratio
9. Define *pharmacodynamic phase*
10. Discuss the importance of structure–activity relationships
11. Discuss the role of drug receptors
12. Discuss the importance of dose–response relationships
13. Describe the importance of pharmacogenetics

KEY TERMS AND DEFINITIONS

Match the following definitions with their terms.

1. _____ A rapid decrease in response to a drug.

2. _____ A drug interaction that occurs from combined drug effects that are greater than if the drugs were given alone.

3. _____ Drug administration in any way other than by the intestine, most commonly by intravenous, intramuscular, or subcutaneous injection.

a. Parenteral
b. Transdermal
c. Inhalation
d. Enteral
e. Lung availability/ systemic availability (L/T ratio)
f. Therapeutic index (TI)

4. _____ Taking a substance, typically in the form of gases, fumes, vapors, mists, aerosols, or dusts, into the body by breathing in.

g. Agonist
h. Synergism
i. Idiosyncratic effect
j. Tachyphylaxis

5. _____ Administration of a drug by use of the intestine.

6. _____ Difference between the minimal therapeutic and toxic concentrations of a drug; the smaller the difference, the greater the chance the drug will be toxic.

7. _____ A chemical or drug that binds to a receptor and creates an effect on the body.

8. _____ An abnormal or unexpected reaction to a drug, other than an allergic reaction, as compared with the predicted effect.

9. _____ The proportion of drug available from the lung, out of the total systemically available drug.

10. _____ Use of a patch on the skin to deliver a drug.

DRUG ADMINISTRATION PHASE

Complete the following questions by writing the correct term in the blank provided.

11. Tablets, capsules, and injectable solutions are examples of _____ _____ forms.

12. Oral, injection, and inhalation are examples of the _____ _____ _____.

13. List the five ways that a drug can be administered along with one example of a common drug formulation.

Route of Administration of Drug

a. _____
b. _____
c. _____
d. _____
e. _____

Common Drug Formulation

a. _____
b. _____
c. _____
d. _____
e. _____

PHARMACOKINETIC PHASE

Complete the following questions in the blank provided.

14. How the drug is absorbed, distributed, metabolized, and eliminated is the _____ phase.

15. How the drug causes an effect in the body is the _____ phase.

16. List the five layers of the lower respiratory tract that a drug must traverse before reaching the bloodstream for distribution into the body.

a. _____

b. _____

c. _____

d. _____

e. _____

Fill in the blank.

17. _____ _____ occurs in the aqueous compartments of the body, such as interstitial spaces or within a cell.

18. _____ _____ occurs across epithelial cells with lipid membranes. For a drug to be distributed in the body, it must cross the many epithelial membranes that have lipid membranes before it reaches the target organ.

19. _____ _____ occurs by special membrane-embedded carrier molecules transporting substances across membranes.

20. _____ is the incorporation of a substance into a cell by a process of membrane engulfment and transport of the substance to the cell interior in vesicles.

21. _____ is the proportion of the drug that reaches the systemic circulation.

22. Drugs that are _____ tend to be well absorbed into the bloodstream and across the blood–brain barrier.

23. List the approximate volume in liters of each of the following major body compartments.

Compartment	Volume (L)
a. Vascular (blood)	_____
b. Interstitial fluid	_____
c. Intracellular fluid	_____
d. Fat (adipose tissue)	_____

24. What two factors can change the *volume of distribution* (V_D)?

    a. _____

    b. _____

25. The main organ for drug metabolism is the _____.

26. List six common pathways for drug metabolism that are considered Phase 1.

    a. _____

    b. _____

    c. _____

    d. _____

    e. _____

    f. _____

27. The major enzyme system in the liver is the _____.

28. List four most important isoenzyme families for drug metabolism.

a. _____

b. _____

c. _____

d. _____

29. Why is it important to know which particular cytochrome P450 (CYP) enzyme metabolizes a drug?

30. If a drug is highly metabolized by the liver, most of the drug's effect will be lost in passing into the liver before it even reaches the general circulation. This clinically important effect is called the _____-_____ effect.

31. List five routes of administration that can bypass the portal venous circulation and avoid the first-pass effect.

a. _____

b. _____

c. _____

d. _____

e. _____

32. The primary site for drug excretion is the _____.

33. _____ is a measure of the ability of the body to rid itself of a drug.

34. The time required for the plasma concentration of a drug to decrease by one-half is called the _____ _____.

35. Why should drugs with a short half-life be given more frequently?

36. In aerosol drug studies that involve bronchodilators, the _____ _____ is often represented, rather than the concentration of the drug.

Using Fig. 2.5 in the textbook, provide the correct answer to the following questions.

37. Which drug would be considered fast acting but of short duration? _____

38. If a person needed a long-acting drug for nighttime, which one would meet the person's needs? _____

39. Which bronchodilator drug would be useful for maintenance therapy and has a duration of action of 4 to 6 hours? _____

Pharmacokinetic Phase
After each question, provide the correct answer(s) or fill in the blank(s).

40. What is the difference between a local drug effect and a systemic drug effect?

41. Give an example of a drug that causes a local effect and a drug that causes a systemic effect.

42. What percentage of an inhaled aerosol is swallowed?

43. What percentage of an inhaled aerosol reaches the lungs?

44. How much aerosol impacts in the mouth and contributes to the amount reaching the stomach?

45. What can be said about lung absorption if the the first-pass metabolism is high?

46. Lung availability/total systemic availability (L/T) basically tells how efficient _____ delivery is into the lung.

47. List four factors that increase the L/T ratio with inhaled drugs.

    a. _____

    b. _____

    c. _____

    d. _____

Complete the following question by writing the correct term in the blank provided.

48. What are *receptors*? _____.

49. What effect does albuterol have on heart rate?

50. The relationship between the chemical structure of a drug and its clinical effect or activity is termed the _____.

51. List the mechanisms of drug receptor action that form the basis for the effects of two drug classes used in respiratory care.

52. List the four mechanisms for transmembrane signaling. Give an example of each.

    a. _____

    b. _____

    c. _____

    d. _____

53. What type of receptors mediate bronchodilation and bronchoconstriction in the airways in response to endogenous stimulation by the neurotransmitters epinephrine and acetylcholine?

54. What term used to describe G proteins with a family of guanine nucleotide–binding proteins with a three-part structure?

55. The body's response to a drug is directly proportional to the drug's _____.

56. The _____ _____ of a drug is the greatest response that can be produced by the drug, so that even at a higher dose, no further response will occur.

57. Which drug is more potent? Drug A (median effective dose [ED_{50}] = 10 mg) or drug B (ED_{50} = 6 mg)?

58. The TI of Drug A is 3, and the TI of Drug B is 50. Which drug is safer?

59. A drug that binds to a receptor (affinity) and causes a response (efficacy) is called a(n) _____.

60. What is the difference between a full agonist and a partial agonist?

Define the following terms.
61. Chemical antagonism

62. Functional antagonism

63. Competitive antagonism

64. _____ _____ refers to when two drugs work against one another. For example, Drug A causes bronchodilation, and Drug B causes bronchoconstriction.

65. A special case of synergism, in which one drug has no effect but can increase the activity of the other drug, is an example of _____.

66. A drug that has the opposite effect, an unusual effect, or no effect compared with the effect it is supposed to have is said to be _____.

67. The term _____ describes an allergic or immune-related response to a drug that can be quite serious, even requiring ventilatory support.

68. The term _____ describes a decreasing intensity of response to a drug over time; over time, more of the drug is required to produce the same effect.

69. The term _____ describes a rapid decrease in responsiveness to a drug.

PHARMACOGENETICS

70. Define pharmacogenetics.

71. List three drugs that are used in respiratory and critical care that have been studied in pharmacogenetics.

    a. _____

    b. _____

    c. _____

NATIONAL BOARD FOR RESPIRATORY CARE (NBRC) TESTING QUESTIONS

1. Which of the following describes what a drug does to the body?
   a. Pharmacology
   b. Pharmacokinetics
   c. Pharmacodynamics
   d. Pharmacogenetics

2. Oral, injection, and inhalation are examples of:
   a. Drug dosage forms
   b. Routes of administration
   c. Pharmacokinetics
   d. Drug formulation

3. Which type of drug crosses the blood–brain barrier most easily?
   1. Nonionized
   2. Ionized
   3. Lipid soluble
   4. Water soluble
      a. 1 and 3
      b. 1 and 4
      c. 2 and 3
      d. 2 and 4

4. Which of the following is the main site of drug metabolism?
   a. Kidney
   b. Stomach
   c. Lung
   d. Liver

5. Which of the following is the main site of drug elimination?
   a. Intestine
   b. Stomach
   c. Kidney
   d. Liver

6. If a drug is administered more frequently than the half-life of the drug, which of the following may result?
   a. Synergy
   b. Accumulation
   c. Elimination
   d. Clearance

7. Which of the following drugs will cause a systemic effect in the body when administered?
   1. Oxymetazdine (Afrin)
   2. Zanamivir (Relenza)
   3. Inhaled morphine
   4. Inhaled insulin
      a. 1, 2
      b. 1, 4
      c. 2, 3, 4
      d. 1, 3, 4

8. Inhaled aerosols used in the treatment of pulmonary disease are intended to exert what effect on the lung?
   a. Local
   b. Systemic
   c. Kinetic
   d. Dynamic

9. The drug dose at which 50% of its maximal response occurs is termed the *ED50*. This refers to what aspect of the drug?
   a. Maximal effect
   b. Half-life
   c. Therapeutic index
   d. Bioavailability

10. Which of the following terms is used to describe what happens when an individual experiences less response to a drug over time?
   a. Hypersensitivity
   b. Idiosyncratic
   c. Toxicity
   d. Tolerance

11. For any drug to cause any effect in the body, it must combine with which of the following?
    a. Target organ
    b. Another carrier drug
    c. Receptor
    d. Blood cell

12. When using a metered dose inhaler (MDI), approximately how much aerosol impacts in the mouth and contributes to the amount reaching the stomach?
    a. 70%
    b. 50%
    c. 10%
    d. 2%

13. What term describes the direct chemical interaction between drug and biologic mediator, which inactivates the drug?
    a. Functional antagonism
    b. Chemical antagonism
    c. Competitive antagonism
    d. Direct antagonism

14. Which of the following L/T ratios indicates more effective drug deposition into the lungs?
    a. 0.92
    b. 0.66
    c. 0.41
    d. 0.17

15. Devices for administration of inhaled drugs include which of the following?
    1. MDI
    2. Dry powder inhaler (DPI)
    3. Pneumatic nebulizer
    4. Ultrasonic nebulizer
        a. 1 and 2
        b. 2 and 3
        c. 2, 3, and 4
        d. 1, 2, 3, and 4

16. What could be done to increase the L/T ratio of an inhaled medication?
    a. Instruct the patient to breath fast and in a shallow manner.
    b. Use inhaled drugs with low first-pass metabolism.
    c. Use a reservoir device or holding chamber with an MDI.
    d. Instruct the patient to breathe slowly when using a DPI.

17. Which of the following is a drug that binds to a receptor and causes a response?
    a. Agonist
    b. Efficist
    c. Additive
    d. Antagonist

18. The effect of two drugs' being greater than the sum of the effect of each drug describes _____.
    a. Potentiation
    b. Additive
    c. Double whammy
    d. Synergism

19. The clinical effect of a bronchodilator is the result of which of the following?
    a. Systemic effects
    b. Drug deposition in the airway
    c. Oral absorption of the drug
    d. Systemic absorption through the stomach

20. The well-described variations among patients in their responses to drugs are increasingly traced to hereditary differences. When do these genetic or hereditary drug variations manifest themselves?
   a. When the patient is administered the drug
   b. During genetic testing
   c. During research of specific groups or individuals
   d. When the drug is discontinued

21. A patient being discharged from the hospital has an order for enteral administration of albuterol sulfate. This would indicate the drug is to be delivered by:
   a. Intravenous route
   b. Inhalation
   c. Mouth
   d. Suppository

22. The lower respiratory tract lining presents barriers to drug absorption. This barrier consists of which of the following:
   a. Type I pneumocyte
   b. Type II pneumocyte
   c. Capillary vascular network
   d. Epithelial lining

23. An order has been written for administration of a drug enterally. This indicates the drug can be given in which of the following forms:
   a. Tablet
   b. Patch
   c. Aerosol
   d. Paste

24. A patient needs a concentration of theophylline equaling 15 mg/L. It is determined that it will take a 525-mg dose to achieve this concentration. This dose is referred to as a:
   a. Loading dose
   b. Functional dose
   c. Primary dose
   d. Clinical dose

25. The following are sedative drugs with their plasma half-life indicated.

Drug	Plasma Half-Life (hr)
A	2.0
B	1.7
C	2.5
D	3.0

If you want a sedative that could be given less frequently, you would suggest which of the following?
   a. Drug A
   b. Drug B
   c. Drug C
   d. Drug D

R.E. is a 24-year-old man who has been brought to the emergency room by his wife because he has had a high fever with shaking chills for the past 24 hours. R.E. states that he has had bronchitis for the past couple of weeks. He is complaining of shortness of breath; his respiratory rate is 32 breaths/min; his heart rate is 108 beats/min. Auscultation reveals bilateral crackles in the lower lobes, with bilateral wheezing heard on inspiration. After examining him, both you and the physician agree that R.E. probably has pneumonia and will be admitted to the hospital for treatment. R.E. will need a bronchodilator for the wheezing and antibiotics for the pneumonia.

1. Which route(s) of administration would be best to deliver the bronchodilator and antibiotics? Explain your choices.

2. What drug would be best for his symptom of bilateral wheezing on inspiration?

R.E. has been admitted to the hospital, and it is now day 2 of his hospital stay. He has been receiving albuterol treatments by small volume nebulizer, and he is feeling much better. His respiratory rate is 18 breaths/min; his heart rate is 84 beats/min. The bilateral wheezing has been reduced, and now he has a slight wheeze bilaterally. R.E. comments that a lot of the medicine seems to be going out into the air and that he can taste it in the back of his throat. He asks you how much of the stuff really makes it into his lungs.

3. What do you tell him?

The doctor has ordered albuterol MDI to be used at home. You suggest that R.E. should also use a reservoir device with the MDI. The doctor does not understand why the reservoir device should also be used.

4. What would you tell the doctor?

Ms. Gonzalez has entered the emergency department because of respiratory distress. After an hour of continuous albuterol treatment, a decision has been made to intubate the patient and place her on mechanical ventilation. The physician administers a short-acting neuromuscular paralyzing agent called *succinylcholine* and a mild sedative. The patient is now paralyzed. The respiratory therapist successfully orally intubates the patient and begins hand ventilation with a resuscitation bag attached to the endotracheal tube. After being placed on a mechanical ventilator, the patient is still paralyzed and not breathing on her own over the ventilator set rate. Both the physician and respiratory therapist believe this is a very unusual situation, because succinylcholine is fast acting and the patient should be paralyzed for only a few minutes, after which she should begin spontaneously breathing.

1. What has caused the prolonged paralysis of Ms. Gonzales?

The patient has been on the ventilator for the past 20 minutes, and the patient is still paralyzed.

2. What should the respiratory therapist recommend?

3 Administration of Aerosolized Agents

CHAPTER OUTLINE

Key Terms and Definitions
Physical Principles of Inhaled Aerosol Drugs
Aerosol Generators for Drug Delivery
Selecting an Aerosol Device
Clinical Application of Aerosol Delivery Devices
Age Guidelines for use of Aerosol Devices
Patient–Device Interface
Recommendations for the Covid-19 Pandemic
National Board for Respiratory Care (NBRC) Testing Questions
Case Studies 1 and 2

CHAPTER OBJECTIVES

After answering the following questions, the reader should be able to:

1. Define terms that pertain to administration of aerosol agents
2. Define *aerosol therapy*
3. Select an appropriate aerosol medication nebulizer on the basis of particle size distributions
4. Discuss aerosol particle size and deposition in the lungs
5. Differentiate between the types of aerosol devices
6. Describe the clinical applications of aerosol devices
7. Recommend the use of various aerosol devices

KEY TERMS AND DEFINITIONS

Complete the following questions by writing the answer in the space provided.

1. The amount of solution that remains in the reservoir of a small-volume nebulizer (SVN) once sputtering begins, causing a decrease in nebulization, is called the _____.

2. What is the term used for testing in a laboratory?

3. What is the term used to describe the diameter of a unit-density spherical particle having the same terminal settling velocity as the measured particle?

4. An aerosol generator is also known as a(n) _____.

5. A nontoxic liquefied gas propellant used to administer medication from a metered dose inhaler (MDI) is a

   _____ _____.

6. An add-on device or extension for administration of a drug from an MDI is known as a _____. It describes both a spacer and a valved holding chamber.

21

7. What is the term used to describe the process of particles' depositing out of suspension to remain in the lung?

8. What is the term used to describe the depth within the lung reached by particles?

9. The tendency of aerosol particles to remain in suspension is described as _____.

10. What is the term used for testing done on animals or humans?

11. _____ refers to the size of particles in an aerosol, meaning many different particle sizes are present.

12. _____ refers to the size of particles in an aerosol, meaning the particles are the same sizes.

13. What is the term used to describe particles in an aerosol are the same size?

14. Delivery of aerosol particles in the lung is called _____ _____.

15. What is the term used to describe a suspension of liquid or solid particles in a carrier gas?

PHYSICAL PRINCIPLES OF INHALED AEROSOL DRUGS

Complete the following questions by writing the answer in the space provided.

16. List three indications for the use of aerosol therapy.

    a. _____

    b. _____

    c. _____

17. List four advantages and disadvantages seen with aerosol delivery of drugs.

Advantages	Disadvantages
a. _____	a. _____
b. _____	b. _____
c. _____	c. _____
d. _____	d. _____

18. The particle size of interest for pulmonary applications is in the range of _____ to _____ μm, and the *fine particle fraction* is considered to include particles smaller than _____ μm.

19. What is the term used to describe the particle size above and below which 50% of the mass of the particles is found?

20. What is the term used to describe the most sensitive technique for quantifying the amount of aerosol on each stage?

21. Aerosol particles with an MMAD range of _____ can make it to the lower respiratory tract. This is the appropriate size for the bronchoactive drugs that we use today.

22. What particle size of aerosols is intended for the terminal airways and alveolar region?

23. What particle size of aerosols is intended for the deposition in the upper airways and early airway generations?

24. Why do aerosol particles released into the atmosphere increase in size?

25. What are three factors that influence aerosol deposition in the lung?

    a. _____

    b. _____

    c. _____

26. The settling of aerosol particles in the lung can increase with encouragement of a _____ - _____.

27. Inhaled aerosol drugs not only are heterodisperse in size, but they also readily absorb moisture; in other words, they are _____.

AEROSOL GENERATORS FOR DRUG DELIVERY

28. SVNs can be classified into three categories. These are:

    a. _____

    b. _____

    c. _____

SELECTING AN AEROSOL DEVICE

29. Identify which nebulizer you would choose for the given clinical situation of a patient needing aerosol therapy.

    a. Older patient debilitated and in acute distress: _____

    b. A person who travels extensively: _____

    c. Drug dose may need to be modified based on patient's level of dyspnea: _____

    d. An infant who cannot hold his or her breath: _____

30. List three names also used to refer to a jet nebulizer.

    a. _____

    b. _____

    c. _____

31. Give a brief description of the following types of nebulizers.

    a. Jet nebulizer with a reservoir tube

    b. Nebulizer with a collection bag

c. Breath-enhanced jet nebulizer

d. Breath-actuated jet nebulizer

e. Manual breath-actuated jet nebulizer

32. Circle the correct answer: Because of significant evaporation of aqueous solution in a gas-powered nebulizer, drug solute can become (increasingly/decreasingly) concentrated.

33. How does a mesh nebulizer work?

34. For efficient operation and relatively brief treatments (≤ 5 minutes), a filling volume of _____ is recommended.

35. With a filling volume of 5 mL, the flow rate should be between _____ and _____.

36. An SVN can be powered using either _____ or _____.

37. Explain why a mouthpiece should be used instead of a face mask for aerosol drug administration.

38. Regardless of the type of device interface used during aerosol therapy, how should you instruct your patients to breathe during aerosol therapy?

39. Higher-viscosity antibiotic solutions of gentamicin or carbenicillin require _____-_____ L/min power gas flow rates to produce suitably small aerosol particles for inhalation with some jet nebulizers.

40. Match the following drug to the approved nebulizer.

1. _____ Iloprost
2. _____ Pentamidine
3. _____ Tobramycin
4. _____ Pulmozyme
5. _____ Ribavirin

a. Pari LC
b. ProDose
c. Hudson T Up-draft II
d. Small-particle aerosol generator (SPAG)
e. Marquest Respirgard II

CLINICAL APPLICATION OF AEROSOL DELIVERY DEVICES

41. Dr. Santiago always orders an SVN for his patient receiving aerosol administration. What are three advantages you could explain to him regarding why the patient could benefit from drug delivery with pressurized MDI (pMDI)?

a. _____

b. _____

c. _____

42. Name the types of pMDIs.

    a. _____

    b. _____

    c. _____

43. Why should a reservoir device be used when delivering inhaled corticosteroids?

44. Describe the instructions you would give a patient for the correct use of their Combivent Respimat soft-mist inhaler.

45. If the pMDI has not been used for several days, what should be done to prime the valve?

46. After aerosol administration of a corticosteroid, what should you instruct your patient to do?

47. If you use both a bronchodilator and a corticosteroid, inhale the bronchodilator first and wait _____ to _____ minutes before inhaling the corticosteroid.

48. What is the most common error when using a pMDI?

    _____

49. What would you tell a patient about how to identify the need to clean the pMDI?

50. Describe each of the following accessory devices for use with pMDI.

    a. Reservoir device

    b. Spacer

    c. Valved holding chamber

51. Describe a DPI.

52. What is the flow rate needed to disperse the drug of a DPI?

53. List three categories of DPI inhalers.

    a. _____

    b. _____

    c. _____

54. What is the biggest limitation of DPI performance and device selection.

55. With any DPI, it is absolutely essential that patients not _____ into the device before inhaling; in all devices, including the Diskus, the drug powder is exposed once the device is activated.

Chapter **3** **Administration of Aerosolized Agents**

AGE GUIDELINES FOR USE OF AEROSOL DEVICES

56. Match the following aerosol systems to the appropriate age.

    1. _____ SVN
    2. _____ MDI
    3. _____ MDI with reservoir
    4. _____ MDI with reservoir and mask
    5. _____ MDI with endotracheal tube (ETT)
    6. _____ Breath-actuated MDI
    7. _____ DPI

    a. More than 5 years of age
    b. Neonate or older
    c. More than 4 years old
    d. Up to 2 years old
    e. Up to 4 years old

57. Do lower or higher flow rates provide more effective the aerosol delivery?

PATIENT–DEVICE INTERFACE

58. If a patient is using a pMDI and a DPI, what difference in the force of inhalation would need to be emphasized between the two devices?
    a. pMDI

    _____

    b. DPI

    _____

59. You have a choice between a mouthpiece or a mask. Which would you choose and why?

60. Where should the SVN be placed in a patient receiving mechanical ventilation to improve aerosol delivery?

61. The _____-_____ _____ should be bypassed when delivering aerosolized medication to a patient receiving mechanical ventilation.

62. The use of a less dense gas, such as a _____-_____ mixture, can increase particle deposition.

63. List three variables present when administering aerosol drug by SVN or MDI to intubated, mechanically ventilated patients.

    SVN

    a. _____

    b. _____

    c. _____

    MDI

    a. _____

    b. _____

    c. _____

64. Your patient is receiving mechanical ventilation due to respiratory failure caused by COVID-19. The physician orders albuterol. Explain your nebulizer choice to deliver the medication.

NATIONAL BOARD FOR RESPIRATORY CARE (NBRC) TESTING QUESTIONS

1. Aerosol therapy is used for which of the following purposes?
   1. Humidification of inspired gases
   2. Improving mobilization and clearance of secretions
   3. Augmenting alveolar ventilation
   4. Delivery of medication
      a. 2 and 3 only
      b. 1 and 4 only
      c. 1, 2, and 4 only
      d. 1, 2, and 3 only

2. Which of the following are advantages of delivering medication using the aerosol versus systemic route of administration?
   1. Smaller doses are required.
   2. Onset of action is slower.
   3. Side effects are fewer.
   4. Drug delivery is targeted to the respiratory system.
      a. 1 and 3 only
      b. 2 and 4 only
      c. 1, 3, and 4 only
      d. 2, 3, and 4 only

3. Which particle size is optimal for aerosol deposition in the terminal airways?
   a. More than 10 μm
   b. 5 to 10 μm
   c. 2 to 5 μm
   d. 0.8 to 3 μm

4. Which of the following is a major risk of health care workers during the COVID-19 pandemic?
   a. Exposure from fugitive aerosols
   b. Burnout
   c. Unknown treatment plans for a new respiratory disease
   d. Staffing shortages

5. A type of nebulizer that uses a plate with multiple apertures and moves the medication through a fine mesh is called:
   a. SVN
   b. SPAG
   c. DPI
   d. Vibrating mesh

6. Which of the following aerosol delivery devices requires the patient to be able to generate an inspiratory flow rate of 30 to 90 L/min?
   a. USN
   b. SPAG
   c. MDI
   d. DPI

7. Which of the following is used to deliver the medication delivery in the Respimat inhaler?
   a. CFC
   b. HFA
   c. A tension spring
   d. Compressed gas

8. The greatest loss of drug with use of a SVN is primarily the result of:
   a. Exhaled medication into the atmosphere
   b. Impaction in the mouth
   c. Reduced deep breathing
   d. Drug remaining in the nebulizer

9. The MMAD of aerosol particles that deposit within the nose and mouth is:
   a. More than 10 μm
   b. 2 to 3 μm
   c. 1 to 2 μm
   d. More than 1 μm

10. For an aerosol to affect the lower respiratory tract of a patient with expiratory wheezing, you would want to use an SVN that delivered aerosol particle sizes in the range of:
    a. 10 to 15 μm
    b. 20 to 25 μm
    c. 1 to 5 μm
    d. 0.5 to 1.0 μm

11. What happens to the amount of drug in a nebulizer when diluent is added?
    a. The amount of drug stays the same.
    b. The concentration is tripled.
    c. The volume is reduced.
    d. The concentration is doubled.

12. With a filling volume of 5 mL in an SVN, the flow rate of the nebulizer should be set to:
    a. 4 L/min
    b. 4 to 5 L/min
    c. 6 to 8 L/min
    d. More than 10 L/min

13. When sputtering of the nebulized medication in an SVN occurs, shaking or agitating the SVN will do which of the following to the drug solution delivery?
    a. Increase the volume of drug solution
    b. Decrease the volume of drug solution
    c. Increase the drug solution concentration and delivery of the drug
    d. Have no effect on delivery of the drug solution

14. Which of the following is not a component of an MDI?
    a. Flow rate control
    b. Metering valve
    c. Propellant
    d. Drug

15. To prevent loss of dose when storing an HFA-propelled MDI canister of a drug, you should:
    a. Shake the MDI before storing it
    b. Store the canister in a valve-up position
    c. Give two puffs before storing the canister
    d. Store the canister on its side

16. When instructing a patient in the use of an MDI that delivers corticosteroids, to reduce oropharyngeal impaction of corticosteroids, you would tell the patient:
    a. To use an open mouth technique when inhaling the medication
    b. To use a closed mouth technique when inhaling the medication
    c. To inhale first and then give the puff of medication
    d. To use a spacer device or holding chambe

17. The term used to describe the loss of propellant from the metering valve of an MDI is:
    a. Creaming
    b. Loss of prime
    c. Actuation
    d. Crystallization

18. When instructing a patient in the use of a holding chamber, when should the patient actuate the pMDI?
    a. At the end of inspiration
    b. In the middle of inspiration
    c. Right before inspiration
    d. All of the above are correct related to actuation timing

19. Which of the following statements is true concerning delivery of a medication during mechanical ventilation of a child or adult?
    a. Using an MDI with a spacer device is better than using an SVN.
    b. Using an MDI without a spacer device is better than using an SVN.
    c. An SVN is better than an MDI with a spacer device.
    d. There is no difference between the use of an SVN and MDI with a spacer device.

20. To improve aerosol delivery during mechanical ventilation, an SVN should be placed:
    a. Directly on the endotracheal tube
    b. Between the Y adapter and the endotracheal tube
    c. After the humidifier but as close to the ventilator and away from the circuit Y as possible
    d. Directly behind the heat-moisture exchanger on the inspiratory side of the patient circuit

21. Which of the following aerosol delivery devices could be used for a child 6 months of age and admitted to the emergency department (ED) with a diagnosis of bronchiolitis?
    a. MDI
    b. DPI
    c. SVN
    d. Breath-actuated MDI

22. When administering aerosol agents to a mechanically ventilated patient with a heat-moisture exchanger in place, the respiratory therapist should:
    a. Increase the inspiratory flow rate of the ventilator during the treatment
    b. Bypass the heat-moisture exchanger
    c. Place the aerosol device within 10 cm of the ETT
    d. Only administer the aerosol agent with an SVN

23. The most common error when using a pMDI is:
    a. Failure to coordinate actuation of MDI with inhalation
    b. Too rapid an inspiratory flow
    c. Inadequate shaking of MDI before use
    d. Actuation of MDI at total lung capacity

24. A patient on mechanical ventilation has been ordered to receive four puffs of a corticosteroid inline through the ventilator. How much time should be given between puffs to allow the valve to refill?
    a. 2 seconds
    b. 20 to 30 seconds
    c. 8 seconds
    d. No waiting is needed between puffs

25. A patient has been ordered to receive a bronchodilator and corticosteroid MDI. Which of the following is the correct method of administration of these drugs?
    a. Use the corticosteroid first, followed immediately by the bronchodilator.
    b. Use the corticosteroid first, then wait 20 to 30 seconds, and then use the bronchodilator.
    c. Use the bronchodilator first, followed immediately by the corticosteroid.
    d. Use the bronchodilator first, wait 1 to 2 minutes, and then use the corticosteroid.

Professor Cooke, a 38-year-old female with a history of asthma, presents to the ED with a chief complaint of shortness of breath and coughing. Her respiratory rate is 34 breaths/min, she is wheezing on both inspiration and expiration throughout both lung fields, and she has accessory muscle usage. She is unable to perform a peak expiratory flow rate maneuver. She complains of anxiety and is diaphoretic, her heart rate is 148 beats/min, and her oxygen saturation is 92% on room air. She is coughing up thick, white, foamy secretions. Oxygen is ordered for Professor Cooke by nasal cannula at 2 L/min, as well as aerosol therapy with albuterol.

1. On the basis of this patient's presentation, what would be your recommendation for the choice of aerosol delivery device?

2. What is your rationale for making this selection?

3. The patient has a total medication volume in the nebulizer of 5 mL. What would be the appropriate flow rate to run the nebulizer? What compressed gas would you choose to power the device? Why?

4. When administering the medication nebulizer, what else could be emphasized to the patient that would help increase lung dose?

It is now 48 hours later. The wheezing has subsided considerably and is now heard slightly on expiration. Professor Cooke has a respiratory rate of 22 breaths/min, oxygen saturation is 97% on room air, and her heart rate is 96 beats/min. She states that she is not experiencing shortness of breath and in general is feeling better. The patient has been ordered to receive a pMDI corticosteroid and a pMDI bronchodilator.

5. How would you instruct the patient in the administration of these drugs regarding which one should be given first?

6. Does she need a reservoir device? Why or why not?

7. Professor Cooke has never used a pMDI and would like to know how she would know when the pMDI is close to the last puff.

Timmy is a 13-year-old patient and has been diagnosed with cystic fibrosis (CF). As part of his respiratory therapy, he has been ordered to receive various respiratory medications.

1. You have decided to administer these medications with a manual breath-actuated jet nebulizer. Because the patient has never used this nebulizer before, how would you instruct Timmy on how to use this device?

2. Because Timmy will be using this nebulizer at home, what would you tell him concerning how often to clean the nebulizer and what should be used to clean the nebulizer?

3. What would you tell Timmy is a way to disinfect the nebulizer?

4 Calculating Drug Doses

CHAPTER OUTLINE

Key Terms and Definitions
Systems of Measure
Calculating Doses From Prepared-Strength Solutions
Calculating Doses From Percentage-Strength Solutions
National Board for Respiratory Care (NBRC) Testing Questions
Case Studies 1, 2, and 3

CHAPTER OBJECTIVES

After answering the following questions, the reader should be able to:

1. Define key terms pertaining to calculating drug dose
2. Use the metric system
3. Calculate drug doses using proportions
4. Calculate drug doses using percentage-strength solutions

KEY TERMS AND DEFINITIONS

Complete the following questions by writing the answer in the space provided.

1. The amount of solute in a solution, usually expressed as a percentage, is called the _____.

2. The amount of solute that is in a solution containing 100 parts is the _____.

3. A physically homogeneous mixture of two or more substances is called a(n) _____.

4. A _____ is a substance that is dissolved in a solution.

5. A substance, usually a liquid, that is used to make a solution is called a _____.

6. The amount of drug that is needed, based on a patient's weight, is called _____.

SYSTEMS OF MEASURE

To do drug calculations, you've got to use the metric system. Warm up with a few practice conversions:

7. 51 cm = _____ mm

8. 33 g = _____ mg

9. 24 mL = _____ L

10. 17 m = _____ cm

11. 68 kg = _____ g

12. 2 teaspoons = _____ drops

13. How many drops are in 1.0 mL? _____

14. A physician orders 1 teaspoon of a medication. How many milliliters does this equate to?

15. If a patient drank four cups of water, it would equal _____ fluid ounces.

16. A baby weighing 2500 g would weigh _____ kg.

17. If you had to give 0.001 L of a drug, you could draw it up in a tuberculin syringe because you would only be giving _____ mL of the drug.

18. Levels of drug in the blood typically have units of measurement of _____ /mL.

CALCULATING DOSES FROM PREPARED-STRENGTH SOLUTIONS

19. Drug A comes in 200-mg tablets. A dose of 500 mg/day is prescribed. How many tablets should the patient take?

20. You are ordered to give 6 mg of dextromethorphan hydrobromide. How many milliliters of dextromethorphan hydrobromide should be given?

21. If there is 100 mg of drug in 50 mL of elixir and you want to give a 10-mg dose, how many milliliters of elixir should be given?

22. How many milliliters do you need to give to deliver 650 U of heparin?

23. Insulin has a standard preparation of 1 unit = _____ mg.

24. A mother of a child receiving albuterol syrup has a prepared mixture of 2 mg/5 mL, and the schedule requires 1 mg/kg. How much syrup is needed for a 25-kg child?

25. How many grams is 25 kg? _____

26. If you have 10 mg/1 mL of morphine in an ampoule for injection, how much is needed to give a 2.0-mg dose intravenously?

27. A dosage schedule of a surfactant calls for 4 mL/kg of body weight for a 1200-g newborn infant. How many milliliters of surfactant will you need to administer?

28. A premature newborn weighs 1000 g. What dose of drug is needed that has a prepared strength of 100 mg/5 mL and a dosing schedule of 100 mg/kg?

CALCULATING DOSES FROM PERCENTAGE-STRENGTH SOLUTIONS

Respiratory therapists often calculate drug doses using solutions and percent strength.

29. To achieve a homogeneous solution, a _____ is dissolved in a _____.

30. What percent strength is a 1:100 solution of a drug?

31. How many milligrams of active ingredient are in 5 mL of a 1:250 drug?

32. A patient needs 3 mL of 10% Mucomyst, but only 20% Mucomyst is available. How much 20% Mucomyst should be used?

33. If you have 2.5 mL of a 20% solution and mix it with 2.5 mL of normal saline for a total of 5 mL, what will be the percent solution?

34. Although the definition of percentage strength in solution involves grams or milliliters, the amount of active ingredient in most nebulized drug solutions is in _____.

35. Complete the following medication calculations.

Percent Strength (%)	Drug Amount (mg/mL)
a. 20%	_____
b. _____	100
c. 0.5	_____
d. 0.05	_____

36. Convert from gram to percent strength to mg/mL.

Grams	Percent Strength	Drug Amount (mg/mL)
a. 0.001	0.1	_____
b. 0.002	_____	2
c. _____	0.3	3

37. If you have 2 mL of a 1% solution of a drug, how many milligrams is the active ingredient?

38. What is the amount of active ingredient in 0.5% strength albuterol that has a usual dose of 0.5 mL?

39. Albuterol has 0.5% strength; what is the drug amount in mg/mL?

40. If you have a drug that is available as 2 mg/mL, what is the percent strength?

NATIONAL BOARD FOR RESPIRATORY CARE (NBRC) TESTING QUESTIONS

1. The respiratory therapist is asked to add 1 g of metaproterenol to 100 mL of aqueous solvent. This will result in which of the following concentrations?
   1. 1:1000
   2. 0.01
   3. 1:100
   4. 1%
      a. 1 and 2 only
      b. 2 and 3 only
      c. 3 and 4 only
      d. 1 and 4 only

2. You are asked to administer 1 mL of a 1% solution of a drug to an asthmatic patient. How many milligrams of drug is this?
   a. 1 mg
   b. 10 mg
   c. 100 mg
   d. 1000 mg

3. The physician's order reads, "Administer 5 mg of metaproterenol via small-volume nebulizer (SVN)." How many milliliters of a 1:100 solution should be used?
   a. 0.5
   b. 1
   c. 1.5
   d. 2

4. The respiratory therapist is asked to dilute 100 mL of a 2% solution of beclomethasone to a 1% solution. How many milliliters of water must be added to the original mixture to produce the desired concentration?
   a. 100
   b. 50
   c. 200
   d. 150

5. How many milliliters of water are needed to dilute 10 mL of a 20% solution of acetylcysteine to a 5% concentration?
   a. 40
   b. 60
   c. 50
   d. 20

6. The physician's order reads, "Instill 5 mL 5% NaHCO$_3$ q4h and prn." The pharmacy has 50-mL ampoules of an 8.4% solution. How many milliliters of distilled water must be added to make a 5% solution?
   a. 10
   b. 21
   c. 34
   d. 42

7. The physician's order reads, "Administer 75 mg Decadron via hand-held nebulizer." How many milliliters of a 2.5% solution should you use?
   a. 2.2
   b. 0.5
   c. 3
   d. 1.5

8. The amount of drug that is needed, based on a patient's weight, is called:
   a. Solution
   b. Body weight proportion
   c. Schedule
   d. Active ingredient

9. What is the percent strength of a drug available at 50 mg/mL?
   a. 1
   b. 5
   c. 10
   d. 15

10. The usual dose of albuterol sulfate is 0.5 mL of a 0.5% strength solution. How many milligrams is this?
    a. 5.0
    b. 2.5
    c. 1.25
    d. 0.50

11. Surfactant has been ordered to be delivered to a premature newborn infant weighing 1.2 kg. What dose should be delivered for a dosage schedule of 5 mL/kg of body weight?
    a. 6 mL
    b. 5 mL
    c. 3 mL
    d. 2.5 mL

12. A patient has been administered 2 g of a drug per 100 mL of solution. This would indicate the patient has received which of the following strength solutions?
    a. 3%
    b. 1%
    c. 2%
    d. 0.5%

13. A patient has just completed a walk down the hospital hallway to determine the oxygen saturation during exercise. The patient walked 1500 cm. How many meters did the patient walk?
    a. 1.5
    b. 5
    c. 15
    d. 20

14. A prescription for an oral medication for a 3-year-old child states to give 1 teaspoon every 8 hours. The mother decides to use a syringe to obtain the medication to give a more exact dosage. How many milliliters of drug should be given?
    a. 1
    b. 3
    c. 5
    d. 6

15. A patient needs 0.5 g of a drug every 8 hours. If each tablet contains a strength of 250 mg, how many tablets should the patient take?
    a. 1
    b. 2
    c. 2.5
    d. 1.5

16. A patient in the emergency department (ED) has been ordered to receive Drug A by injection. One ampoule contains 1 mg/mL of Drug A. The order states to give a 0.25-dose subcutaneously. How many milliliters should be administered?
    a. 0.25
    b. 0.50
    c. 1
    d. 1.25

17. A patient admitted for exacerbation of asthma has been ordered to receive albuterol. The order states, "albuterol q4h and prn with 5 mg/mL solution by SVN." As you are giving the treatment, the resident making rounds asks what is the percentage strength of the albuterol. Based on the prescription, the patient is receiving:
    a. 0.1%
    b. 0.5%
    c. 0.25%
    d. 0.4%

18. The _____ of a drug is the amount of solute in a solution, usually expressed as a percentage.
    a. Solution
    b. Solute
    c. Solvent
    d. Strength

19. On a patient's chart, you read that the patient drank two cups of apple juice for breakfast. This would be equal to

    _____ mL.
    a. 64
    b. 100
    c. 220
    d. 480

20. A 3-mL unit dose of albuterol with a percentage strength of 0.083% is available for administration. What should be done so that the usual dose of 2.5 mg is delivered?
    a. Mix the unit dose with 5 mL of normal saline.
    b. Mix 1 mL of the unit dose and 1 mL of normal saline.
    c. Administer all 3 mL of the unit dose to the patient.
    d. Mix the unit dose with 3 mL of normal saline.

CASE STUDY 1

A physician orders Drug B to be delivered by SVN to one of your patients. The drug is available as 20 mg in 2 mL of aqueous solution. What percentage strength are you delivering to your patient? (*Hint:* You're doing a weight-to-volume calculation.)

CASE STUDY 2

A 45-year-old patient is admitted to the intensive care unit with Tylenol overdose. The treatment calls for administration of 6 mL of 20% Mucomyst. Only 10% Mucomyst is available. How much 10% Mucomyst is needed to prepare 6 mL of 20% Mucomyst?

CASE STUDY 3

A 6-year-old child is being discharged from the hospital, and the mother has a medication that has a dropper that is able to measure 1 mL. The prescription calls for the child to receive 0.5 mL of the medication every 6 hours. The mother is concerned that she will not get the medication exact.

1. What should the mother do to ensure an exact amount of drug?

The mother states that she has "measuring spoons" that she uses for baking at home, and she feels they are very accurate. She has a one-half teaspoon measuring spoon that she could use to give her child medication, and this way she wouldn't have to count out the drops.

2. What could you say to the mother concerning using household measuring spoons to administer medication?

5 Central and Peripheral Nervous Systems

CHAPTER OBJECTIVES

After answering the following questions, the reader should be able to:

1. Define key terms pertaining to the central and peripheral nervous systems
2. Classify the branches of the nervous system
3. Differentiate among the *central, peripheral,* and *autonomic nervous systems*
4. Discuss the use of *neurotransmitters*
5. Explain in detail the difference between the *parasympathetic* and *sympathetic* branches of the nervous system
6. Differentiate between the effects of *cholinergic* and *anticholinergic agents* on the nervous system
7. Differentiate between the effects of *adrenergic* and *antiadrenergic agents* on the nervous system
8. Discuss the various receptors in the airways
9. Differentiate among *nonadrenergic, noncholinergic inhibitory,* and *excitatory* nerves

KEY TERMS AND DEFINITIONS

Complete the following questions by writing the correct term in the blanks provided.

1. The portion of the nervous system that includes the brain and spinal cord, controlling voluntary and involuntary acts,

    is called the _____ _____ _____.

2. The portion of the nervous system that is outside the central nervous system and includes the sensory, sympathetic,

    and parasympathetic nerves is known as the _____ _____ _____.

3. Signals that are transmitted *from* the brain and spinal cord are called _____.

4. Signals that are transmitted *to* the brain and spinal cord are called _____.

5. The neurotransmitter used at postganglionic sympathetic nerve sites is _____.

6. The neurotransmitter used in the transmission of nerve impulses in the parasympathetic nervous system is

    _____. It is destroyed by cholinesterase.

7. A drug stimulating a receptor for norepinephrine or epinephrine is called _____.

8. A drug blocking a receptor for acetylcholine is called _____.

9. An agent causing stimulation of parasympathetic nervous system sites is called _____.

10. An agent that blocks the effect of the sympathetic nervous system is called _____.

11. An agent that blocks the effect of the parasympathetic nervous system is called _____.

12. An agent that stimulates the sympathetic nervous system is called _____.

THE NERVOUS SYSTEM

Complete the following questions by writing the correct term in the blank provided.

13. What are the two major control systems in the body?

14. The nervous system is divided into two parts. List each part.

    a. _____

    b. _____

15. Which nervous system contains the parasympathetic and sympathetic nervous systems?

16. The parasympathetic branch arises from which part of the spinal cord?

17. The sympathetic branch arises from the _____ portion of the spinal cord.

18. Because sympathetic fibers innervate the adrenal medulla, after sympathetic activation there is a release of _____ into the bloodstream.

19. List three characteristics of both the parasympathetic and sympathetic nervous systems.

    Parasympathetic nervous system

    a. _____

    b. _____

    c. _____

    Sympathetic nervous system

    a. _____

    b. _____

    c. _____

20. Give an example of when you would expect your sympathetic nervous system to activate.

Note: To understand medications, you need to understand neurotransmitters.

21. Neurotransmitters control what type of impulses?

22. The neurotransmitter located in skeletal muscle, the parasympathetic nervous system terminal nerve sites, and all ganglionic synapses is _____.

23. The autonomic nervous system is generally thought to be what kind of system?

24. The neurotransmitter conducting the nerve impulse at smooth muscle sites is _____.

25. Norepinephrine and sympathetic transmission are terminated by _____, _____, and _____.

26. Match each of the following terms with its corresponding definition.

1. _____ Sympathomimetic	a. Agent blocking sympathetic nervous system
2. _____ Adrenergic	b. Agent stimulating parasympathetic nervous system
3. _____ Parasympatholytic	c. Agent blocking epinephrine receptor
4. _____ Anticholinergic	d. Agent blocking acetylcholine receptor
5. _____ Antiadrenergic	e. Agent stimulating sympathetic nervous system
6. _____ Parasympathomimetic	f. Agent stimulating acetylcholine receptor
7. _____ Cholinergic	g. Agent blocking parasympathetic nervous system
8. _____ Sympatholytic	h. Agent stimulating epinephrine receptor

Parasympathetic Branch

27. Fill in the changes that occur with parasympathetic (cholinergic) stimulation:

a. Heart: _____

b. Bronchial smooth muscle: _____

c. Exocrine glands: _____

28. Two additional terms used to refer to stimulation of receptor sites by acetylcholine are

a. _____, because of the effect of nicotine, and

b. _____, because of the effect of muscarine.

29. How will the administration of a muscarinic drug effect airway secretions?

30. A parasympathomimetic effect is the same as a _____ effect, and a parasympatholytic effect is the same as a _____ effect.

31. The term *nicotinic* refers to cholinergic receptors on ganglia and at the _____.

CHOLINERGIC AND ANTICHOLINERGIC AGENTS

Complete the following questions by writing the answer in the space provided.

32. Name a direct-acting cholinergic drug that is used to assess the degree of airway reactivity in suspected asthmatic patients: _____

33. An indirect-acting cholinergic agent that is short acting and a useful diagnostic agent for myasthenia gravis is:

    a. Generic name _____

    b. Brand name _____

34. Parasympatholytics and neuromuscular blocking agents block acetylcholine receptors and are therefore _____ agents.

35. Name an antihistamine drug with an anticholinergic effect, commonly used to prevent motion sickness.

36. List four uses of a parasympatholytic or antimuscarinic agent such as atropine.

    a._____

    b. _____

    c._____

    d. _____

Sympathetic Branch

37. Circle the correct answer: Stimulation of the heart should (increase/decrease) cardiac output.

38. The neurotransmitter at the terminal nerve sites in the sympathetic branch of the autonomic nervous system is _____.

39. The following are sympathomimetic drugs. Fill in their uses.

Drug	Uses
Epinephrine	a. _____
Albuterol	b. _____
Salmeterol	c. _____
Dopamine	d. _____

40. List two types of sympathetic receptors.

    a. _____

    b. _____

41. Stimulation of α_1 receptors causes _____.

42. Stimulation of β_1 receptors increases the _____ and _____ _____ _____ of cardiac smooth muscle.

43. Stimulation of β_2 receptors causes _____ and _____ muscle relaxation.

44. Which receptors (α_1, β_1, or β_2) would be best to stimulate if a patient had a runny nose?

45. Which receptors (α_1, β_1, or β_2) would be best to stimulate to give relief to a patient in the midst of an asthma attack?

46. The chemical found in the brain that is a precursor of norepinephrine and stimulates both α_1 and α_2 receptors is called

    _____.

NEURAL CONTROL OF LUNG FUNCTION

Complete the following questions by writing the correct term in the blank provided.

47. Although no direct sympathetic innervation of airway smooth muscle occurs, the sympathetic nervous system controls smooth muscle tone by circulating _____.

48. Epinephrine acts on both _____ and _____ receptors, whereas norepinephrine acts primarily on _____ receptors.

49. β agonists, distributed from the trachea to terminal bronchioles, cause _____ of small airways.

50. What receptor type are the adrenergic receptors in the lung?

51. Are β_1 or α receptors located in the alveolar walls and lung periphery?

52. True or False: The α receptors are located equally throughout large and small airways and are less abundant than β receptors.

53. The lungs receive their blood supply from both the _____ and the _____ circulations.

54. Pulmonary circulation is innervated by both the _____ _____ _____ and the _____ _____ nervous systems.

55. Arterial (bronchial) circulation is innervated mostly by which nervous system?

56. Bronchial submucosal glands are innervated by which nervous systems?

57. When bronchial mucosal glands are stimulated, what happens to mucus production?

58. Airway smooth muscle responds to circulating _____ by means of α receptors.

59. Submucosal glands have which types of receptors?

60. The lungs are innervated by which nerve that enters the lungs at the hilum and innervates intrapulmonary airways?

61. What is the bronchial smooth muscle response to stimulation of the vagus nerve?

62. What will happen to submucosal gland secretions when the vagus nerve is stimulated?

63. Three muscarinic receptor sites are present in the lung. Which of these, M_1, M_2, or M_3, is located on submucosal glands and airway smooth muscle? _____

64. Muscarinic receptor M_3 is located on blood vessels and causes the release of an endothelial-derived relaxant factor that produces what effect of both the bronchial and pulmonary vasculature?

65. Evidence indicates a branch of nerves other than adrenergic or cholinergic that cause bronchodilation. These nerves are called _____ and _____ system.

66. Inhibitory effects on airway smooth muscle cause bronchodilation and may be mediated by the neurotransmitter _____ or by _____ _____.

67. Excitatory effects such as bronchoconstriction are produced by afferent sensory fibers that have _____ _____ as a neurotransmitter.

NATIONAL BOARD FOR RESPIRATORY CARE (NBRC) TESTING QUESTIONS

1. The sympathetic nervous system is part of which of the following?
   a. Central nervous system
   b. Parasympathetic nervous system
   c. Autonomic nervous system
   d. Endocrine system

2. Which branch of the nervous system controls daily functions, such as digestion and bladder control?
   a. Central nervous system
   b. Parasympathetic nervous system
   c. Sympathetic nervous system
   d. Edocrine system

3. Which of the following describes a drug that stimulates the sympathetic nervous system?
   a. Parasympathomimetic
   b. Parasympatholytic
   c. Sympathomimetic
   d. Sympatholytic

4. Which of the following describes the autonomic nervous system?
   a. Sends impulses from the brain to the neuroeffector sites
   b. Sends impulses from the periphery to the brain and spinal cord
   c. Is exemplified by the knee-jerk reaction
   d. Is an afferent system

5. Which of the following describes a drug that blocks a receptor for acetylcholine?
   a. Cholinergic
   b. Anticholinergic
   c. Adrenergic
   d. Antiadrenergic

6. Sympathetic nervous system stimulation results in which of the following?
   a. Decreased blood pressure
   b. Mental stimulation
   c. Decreased heart rate
   d. Bronchoconstriction

7. Which two enzymes inactivate catecholamines?
   a. TDH and BHG
   b. COTN and MNM
   c. AchE and TKO
   d. COMT and MAO

8. Stimulation of which of the following receptors results in vasoconstriction?
   a. α
   b. β_1
   c. β_2
   d. γ

9. Epinephrine accomplishes which of the following?
   a. Stimulates primarily α receptors
   b. Stimulates primarily β receptors
   c. Stimulates α and β receptors equally
   d. Stimulates neither α nor β receptors

10. Blood flow to the lung is supplied by which of the following?
    1. Pulmonary circulation
    2. Vagal circulation
    3. Bronchial circulation
    4. Parasympathetic circulation
       a. 1 and 4 only
       b. 2 and 3 only
       c. 1 and 3 only
       d. 2 and 4 only

11. Bronchodilation most likely occurs as a result of stimulation of which receptor?
    a. α_1
    b. α_2
    c. β_1
    d. β_2

12. Relaxation of airway smooth muscle should *not* occur with which of the following?
    a. Stimulation of the nonadrenergic inhibitory nerves
    b. Use of a cholinergic agent
    c. Use of a sympathomimetic
    d. Use of a parasympatholytic

13. A drug that stimulates the parasympathetic nervous system will cause which of the following?
    a. Slower heart rate
    b. Bronchodilation
    c. Reduced secretions
    d. Thicker secretions

14. Which of the following are sympathomimetic or adrenergic agonists?
    1. Epinephrine
    2. Propranolol
    3. Albuterol
    4. Salmeterol
        a. 1 and 4 only
        b. 1, 2, and 3 only
        c. 1, 3, and 4 only
        d. 2, 3, and 4 only

15. Adrenergic receptors in the lungs are:
    a. All α_1
    b. All β_1
    c. All β_2
    d. α_1 and β_2

16. Bronchial submucosal glands are innervated by:
    a. Parasympathetic nervous system
    b. Sympathetic nervous system
    c. Both parasympathetic and sympathetic nervous systems
    d. Edocrnine system

17. The nerve that innervates the lungs and enters at the hilum is the:
    a. Phrenic
    b. Pulmonic
    c. Glossopharyngeal
    d. Vagus

18. Stimulation of β_1 receptors of cardiac smooth muscle will cause which of the following?
    1. Increased heart rate
    2. Reduced cardiac output
    3. Coronary artery constriction
    4. Increased force of contraction
        a. 1 and 3 only
        b. 1 and 4 only
        c. 1, 2, and 3 only
        d. 2, 3, and 4 only

19. A patient has just received a medication and is now experiencing relief from an exacerbation of asthma. Based on this information, which of the following agonists was given?
    a. α_1
    b. β_1
    c. α_2
    d. β_2

20. Which of the following would be a sympathomimetic effect of epinephrine?
    a. Bronchodilation
    b. Miosis
    c. Vasodilation
    d. Bradycardia

21. A direct-acting cholinergic agent used to help diagnose asthma is:
    a. Mestinon
    b. Methacholine
    c. Pilocarpine
    d. Tensilon

22. Which of the following drugs is a muscarinic that increases airway secretions?
    a. Neostigmine
    b. Epinephrine
    c. Atropine
    d. Albuterol

23. To help reduce airway secretions during surgery, which of the following drugs is given before surgery in patients?
    a. Tensilon
    b. Epinephrine
    c. Atropine
    d. Pilocarpine

24. Which of the following muscarinic receptor sites found in the lung is located on submucosal glands and smooth muscle?
    a. M_1
    b. M_2
    c. M_3
    d. M_5

25. To relieve nasal congestion, you would purchase a medication that has which of the following drug ingredients?
    a. Ephedrine
    b. Amphetamine
    c. Albuterol
    d. Salmeterol

CASE STUDY 1

Methacholine is an inhaled parasympathomimetic agent used in bronchial challenge tests to determine the degree of airway reactivity in asthmatic individuals.

1. What is the parasympathetic effect?

2. Explain how methacholine works to detect the degree of airway reactivity?

CASE STUDY 2

A 49-year-old woman has entered the emergency department (ED) with complaints of weakness involving her face, eyes, and arms. The patient explains that she has experienced blurred vision that comes and goes, and also her eyelids are drooping. She further states that she has problems swallowing, and she sometimes chokes when swallowing liquids. Additionally, she notes that recently she has had difficulty lifting light objects. After the ED doctor consults with a neurologist, it is concluded that she may have myasthenia gravis, and the decision is made to do an edrophonium (Tensilon) test.

1. What is the purpose of administering edrophonium (Tensilon) to this patient?

2. Why is this drug classified as an indirect-acting cholinergic agonist?

3. Why is edrophonium used?

4. Tensilon can be administered by two routes, either pill or intravenously. Which would be the best route of administration for this patient? Explain your answer.

5. What indirect-acting cholinergic maintenance drug is prescribed for muscle stimulation for patients with myasthenia gravis?

6. What are two undesirable effects associated with the use of either of these indirect cholinergic maintenance drugs?

    a. _____

    b. _____

7. Prior to medications being prescribed, the physician needs to make sure the test for myasthenia gravis was not a false-positive. What additional test can be done?

Adrenergic (Sympathomimetic) Bronchodilators

CHAPTER OUTLINE

Key Terms and Definitions
Clinical Indications for Adrenergic Bronchodilators
Long-Acting β-Adrenergic Agents
Mode of Action
Routes of Administration
Adverse Side Effects
β-Agonist Controversy
Respiratory Care Assessment of β-Agonist Therapy
National Board of Respiratory Care (NBRC) Testing Questions
Case Studies 1 and 2

CHAPTER OBJECTIVES

After answering the following questions, the reader should be able to:

1. Define *sympathomimetic*
2. Define *adrenergic*
3. List all currently available β-adrenergic agents used in respiratory therapy
4. Differentiate between the specific adrenergic agents and formulations
5. Describe the mechanism of action for each specific adrenergic agent and formulation
6. Describe the route of administration available for β agonists
7. Discuss adverse effects of β agonists
8. Clinically assess β-agonist therapy

Chapter 6 is of particular importance because inhaled adrenergic bronchodilators represent the medications most commonly administered by respiratory therapists.

KEY TERMS AND DEFINITIONS

Complete the following questions by writing the correct answer in the blank provided.

1. What is the name of the enzyme that produces the opposite reaction of that produced by cyclic adenosine monophosphate (cAMP), and causes bronchoconstriction?

2. What produces effects similar to those of the sympathetic nervous system?

3. What is narrowing of the airways resulting from contraction of smooth muscle called?

4. A group of similar compounds having sympathomimetic action and mimicking the actions of epinephrine is the

   _____.

5. An agent that stimulates sympathetic nervous fibers and allows relaxation of smooth muscle in the airway is a

   _____ _____.

6. A drug that exhibits pharmacologic activity once it is converted, inside the body, to its active form is called a

   _____.

7. _____ stimulation causes vasoconstriction and a vasopressor effect in the upper airway, which provides decongestion.

8. What receptor when stimulated causes increased myocardial conductivity, heart rate, and contractile force?

9. Wht is long-term desensitization of β receptors to β_2 agonists, caused by a reduction in the number of β receptors called?

10. _____ stimulation causes relaxation of bronchial smooth muscle with some inhibition of inflammatory mediator release and stimulation of mucociliary clearance.

11. _____ _____ refers to the increasing incidence of asthma morbidity, and especially asthma mortality, despite advances in the understanding of asthma and availability of improved drugs to treat asthma.

12. _____ _____ is a nucleotide-produced β_2-receptor stimulation that causes relaxation of bronchial smooth muscle.

13. What are the results of α and β_1 receptor stimulation?

14. List three effects that β_2-specific drugs produce.

   a. _____

   b. _____

   c. _____

CLINICAL INDICATIONS FOR ADRENERGIC BRONCHODILATORS

15. What is the general indication for adrenergic bronchodilators?

16. List two short-acting adrenergic bronchodilators.

   a. _____

   b. _____

17. List five long-acting adrenergic bronchodilators.

    a. _____

    b. _____

    c. _____

    d. _____

    e. _____

18. What is the major difference between the indication for short-acting agents compared with long-acting agents?

19. List three indications for administration of racemic epinephrine.

    a. _____

    b. _____

    c. _____

20. Put a check mark next to the symptoms that may occur with administration of a catecholamine:

    a. Tachycardia: _____

    b. Bronchoconstriction: _____

    c. Elevated blood pressure: _____

    d. Bronchodilation: _____

    e. Increased urine output: _____

    f. Relaxation of skeletal muscle blood vessels: _____

21. Why shouldn't catecholamines be given orally?

22. What enzyme metabolizes epinephrine?

23. Explain how catecholamines were made more β_2 specific.

24. List five ways in which albuterol can be delivered.

    a. _____

    b. _____

    c. _____

    d. _____

    e. _____

25. List three trade names for albuterol that a respiratory therapist can deliver via inhalation.

    a. _____

    b. _____

    c. _____

26. What is a prodrug?

27. List the three strengths of nebulized solutions of levalbuterol that are available.

    a. _____

    b. _____

    c. _____

28. The brand name for levalbuterol is _____.

29. List eight effects and characteristics of the (S)-isomer of albuterol.

    a. _____

    b. _____

    c. _____

    d. _____

    e. _____

    f. _____

    g. _____

    h. _____

30. Fill in the blanks regarding levalbuterol (Xopenex):

a. Onset of action: _____

b. Peak effect: _____

c. Duration of effect: _____

d. Receptor preference: _____

e. Routes available: _____

LONG-ACTING β-ADRENERGIC AGENTS

31. Fill in the chart regarding long-acting bronchodilator agents.

Generic Name	Brand Name	Receptor Preference	Adult Dosage	Time Course (Onset, Peak, Duration)
Salmeterol				
Formoterol				
Arformoterol				
Olodaterol				

32. VoSpire ER is an extended-release form of _____ that has an extended activity up to _____ hours.

33. List four points that should be noted in the clinical use of long-acting agents because of their differences from shorter-acting β agonists.

a.

b.

c.

d.

34. Because of the ongoing safety concerns regarding long-acting β_2 agonists, the U.S. Food and Drug Administration (FDA) is now requiring changes on how long-acting β_2 agonists are used in the treatment of asthma. List five of these requirements.

a.

b.

c.

d.

e.

MODE OF ACTION

35. Match the following modes of action with the type of receptor stimulation:

1. _____ Upper airway vasoconstriction

2. _____ Relaxation of bronchial smooth muscle

3. _____ Stimulation of mucociliary clearance

4. _____ Increased heart rate

5. _____ Decongestion in the nasal passages

6. _____ Increased contractile force of the heart

7. _____ Some inhibition of inflammatory mediator release

a. α-Receptor stimulation
b. β_1-Receptor stimulation
c. β_2-Receptor stimulation

ROUTES OF ADMINISTRATION

36. The following is a list of routes of administration. Indicate for each route whether it is currently available *(Y for Yes)* or not available *(N for No)* for β-adrenergic bronchodilators:
a. metered dose inhaler (MDI): _____
b. dry powder inhaler (DPI): _____
c. Tablet: _____
d. Syrup: _____
e. Nebulizer solution: _____
f. Parenteral: _____
g. Suppository: _____

37. List five reasons why inhalation is the preferred route of administration of a β-adrenergic drug:

    a. _____

    b. _____

    c. _____

    d. _____

    e. _____

38. Why must catecholamines be given via inhalation?

39. List five advantages of the oral inhalation route in administering β agonists.

    a. _____

    b. _____

    c. _____

    d. _____

    e. _____

ADVERSE SIDE EFFECTS

40. Adverse side effects can occur with β agonists. Name three side effects.

    a. _____

    b. _____

    c. _____

41. What does *tolerance* mean?

42. A fall in the partial pressure of arterial oxygen (Pao_2) has been noted with newer β agonists, such as albuterol and salmeterol. Explain why.

43. Despite our increased understanding of asthma and the availability of improved drug treatment, asthma morbidity and mortality seem to be increasing. The role that β_2 medications play in this phenomenon is unclear. List five possible reasons suggested by the literature.

a.

b.

c.

d.

e.

RESPIRATORY CARE ASSESSMENT OF β-AGONIST THERAPY

44. *Circle True or False in the following statements:*
    a. True or False: A peak flow meter can be used to assess the reversibility of airflow obstruction at the bedside.
    b. True or False: The respiratory care practitioner should assess breathing rate and pattern and breath sounds before and after the completion of treatment.
    c. True or False: Potassium can decrease, and blood glucose can increase with the use of continuous nebulization of a β agonist.
    d. True or False: When educating a patient about asthma, it should be emphasized that only β agonists are needed to prevent severe asthma episodes.
    e. True or False: Patient education should include the correct use of aerosol devices, as well as assembly and cleaning of devices.
    f. True or False: When assessing a patient to determine the benefit of long-acting β agonists, the respiratory care practitioner should assess nocturnal symptoms, number of exacerbations, unscheduled clinic or hospital visits, and days of absence from work related to symptoms.

NATIONAL BOARD OF RESPIRATORY CARE (NBRC) TESTING QUESTIONS

1. β_2-Receptor stimulation has which of the following effects?
    a. Mucous gland hypertrophy
    b. Bronchial smooth muscle relaxation
    c. Decreased peripheral blood flow
    d. Increased pulmonary blood flow

2. Catecholamines do which of the following?
   a. Mimic the action of catechol
   b. Mimic the action of epinephrine
   c. Have a prolamine nucleus
   d. Are α inhibitors

3. Which of the following describes catecholamines?
   a. Long acting
   b. Slow onset
   c. Useful for asthma maintenance therapy
   d. Inactivated by catechol-*O*-methyltransferase (COMT)

4. Catecholamines are unsuitable for which route of administration?
   a. Intravenous
   b. Inhalation
   c. Oral
   d. Subcutaneous

5. Vilanterol is an example of which type of adrenergic bronchodilator?
   a. Catecholamine
   b. Resorcinol
   c. Saligenin
   d. Sustained release

6. Which of the following drugs is a long-acting bronchodilator?
   a. Levalbuterol
   b. Epinephrine
   c. Indacterol
   d. Proventil

7. Which of the following strengths are available for nebulization of levalbuterol?
   1. 0.31 mg
   2. 0.63 mg
   3. 1.25 mg
   4. 2.50 mg
      a. 1 and 2 only
      b. 3 and 4 only
      c. 1, 2, and 3 only
      d. 2, 3, and 4 only

8. Perforomist can be given as a liquid nebulization and is currently approved only for:
   a. Exercise-induced asthma
   b. Asthma with nocturnal sleeping problems
   c. COPD
   d. Pulmonary fibrosis

9. Which of the following catecholamines or catecholamine derivatives lasts the longest?
   a. Albuterol
   b. Racemic epinephrine
   c. Metaproterenol
   d. Salmeterol

10. Which of the following diseases is likely to respond well to adrenergic bronchodilators?
    1. Asthma
    2. Cystic fibrosis
    3. Chronic bronchitis
    4. Pulmonary fibrosis
        a. 1 and 2 only
        b. 3 and 4 only
        c. 1, 2, and 3 only
        d. 2, 3, and 4 only

11. Which of the following drugs can be administered both subcutaneously and by inhalation to treat asthma exacerbation?
    a. Acetylcholine
    b. Norepinephrine
    c. Epinephrine
    d. Dopamine

12. Which of the following is a form of single-isomer albuterol?
    a. Salmeterol
    b. Levalbuterol
    c. Olodaterol
    d. Arformoterol

13. In relation to bronchodilators, "rescue" agents refer to:
    a. Short-acting agents
    b. Long-acting agents
    c. Controllers
    d. Prodrugs

14. Which of the following are saligenins?
    1. Terbutaline
    2. Epinephrine
    3. Levalbuterol
    4. Albuterol
        a. 1 and 2 only
        b. 3 and 4 only
        c. 1, 2, and 3 only
        d. 2, 3, and 4 only

15. Which of the following are short-acting bronchodilators?

16. What strength of racemic epinephrine is used for nebulization?
    a. 2.25%
    b. 1%
    c. 3%
    d. 1.25%

17. Albuterol can be delivered via a variety of routes of administration, including:
    1. DPI
    2. Ointment
    3. Nebulizer solution
    4. MDI
        a. 1 and 3 only
        b. 2 and 3 only
        c. 2, 3, and 4 only
        d. 1, 3, and 4 only

18. Which of the following are side effects associated with β agonists?
    1. Tremor
    2. Palpitations
    3. Bradycardia
    4. Headache
        a. 1 and 2 only
        b. 2 and 4 only
        c. 1, 3, and 4 only
        d. 2, 3, and 4 only

19. Exposure to which of the following readily inactivates catecholamines?
    a. Oxygen
    b. Saline
    c. Light
    d. Air

20. The only pure (R)-isomer of racemic albuterol that is a short-acting bronchodilator available in the U.S. market is:
    a. Xopenex
    b. Severent
    c. Proventil
    d. Brovana

21. Formoterol, like salmeterol, has a long-lasting bronchodilating effect up to _____ hours of duration.
    a. 6
    b. 5
    c. 12
    d. 23

22. Aformoterol is a long-acting β_2-selective agonist that is approved by the FDA as:
    a. Stovana
    b. Afrobrovana
    c. Brovona
    d. R-Stovana

23. National guidelines recommend the introduction of a long-acting β agonist in step 3 care of asthma when which of the following conditions exists?
    a. Asthma controlled by short-acting β agonists
    b. Asthma not controlled by lower doses of anti-inflammatory medicine
    c. Asthma not controlled by higher doses of anti-inflammatory medicine
    d. Asthma not controlled by short-acting β agonist and high doses of anti-inflammatory medicine

24. Which of the following statements regarding the drop in Pa_{O_2} after bronchodilator administration by inhalation is true?
    1. It occurs because of ventilation-perfusion mismatch.
    2. The drop is physiologically significant.
    3. The drop is statistically significant.
    4. The drop in oxygen saturation (Sa_{O_2}) is minimal.
        a. 2 only
        b. 1 and 3 only
        c. 1, 3, and 4 only
        d. 2, 3, and 4 only

25. The general indication for adrenergic bronchodilators is to:
    a. Reduce the consistency of mucus
    b. Reduce inflammation
    c. Reduce blood flow to target organs
    d. Reverse or lessen the degree of airflow obstruction

26. Epinephrine is a potent catecholamine bronchodilator; in addition, what other receptors does it effect?
    a. α only
    b. β_1 only
    c. α and β_1
    d. β_2 only

27. A pediatric patient has stridor and has been diagnosed with croup. To help reduce the swelling in the upper airway, which drug would be most beneficial?
    a. Racemic epinephrine
    b. Arformoterol
    c. Albuterol
    d. Levalbuterol

28. Albuterol has which of the following actions?
    1. Duration up to 8 to 12 hours
    2. β_2 preferential
    3. Peak effect within 30 to 60 minutes
    4. Can be delivered by mouth
        a. 1 and 2 only
        b. 2 and 3 only
        c. 1, 2, and 3 only
        d. 2, 3, and 4 only

29. This drug is used for prevention of acute exercise-induced bronchospasm in adults and children older than 5 years of age:
    a. Salmeterol
    b. Levalbuterol
    c. Albuterol
    d. Formoterol

30. The National Asthma Education and Prevention Program (NAEPP) Expert Panel Report 3 (EPR 3) Guidelines on Asthma consider salmeterol to be which of the following types of drug?
    a. Controller
    b. Rescue
    c. Reliever
    d. Short term and rescue

31. Asthmatic patients must be educated that the use of β agonists will:
    a. Treat inflammation
    b. Treat poor pulmonary blood flow
    c. Be used as a rescue medication for exacerbations of their asthma
    d. Prevent the use of medication to treat aggressive asthma

32. Which of the following is a reason why inhalation is the preferred route of administration of a β-adrenergic drug?
    a. Slow onset
    b. Larger dose required compared with the oral route
    c. Reduced side effects
    d. Reduced lung availability/total systemic availability (L/T) ratio

33. A practical approach to optimal drug dosing in a patient brought to the emergency department with severe airway

    obstruction, and who does not respond to intermittent nebulizer treatments after 1 hour, would be _____

    _____ of β agonists.
    a. Increasing dosage
    b. Oral administration
    c. Subcutaneous injection
    d. Continuous nebulization

34. A respiratory therapist tells the physician that he is measuring the bronchodilating effect of a β agonist. The therapist would be:
    a. Determining the reaction of the airway by cold air introduction
    b. Determining the reaction of the airway by the amount of wheezing produced by methacholine challenge
    c. Measuring airflow changes by measuring forced expiratory volume at 1 second (FEV_1)
    d. Determining the reaction of the airway by introduction of histamine

35. Which of the following would be used to assess reversibility of airflow obstruction?
    1. Peak flow meter
    2. Incentive spirometer
    3. Portable spirometry
    4. Pulse oximetry
        a. 1 and 3 only
        b. 2 and 4 only
        c. 1, 3, and 4 only
        d. 2, 3, and 4 only

36. To assess the effectiveness of long-acting β agonists, you would do which of the following?
    a. Assess ongoing lung function by peak expiratory flow
    b. Send patient questionnaire every 6 weeks
    c. Obtain blood culture every 6 months
    d. Assess ongoing lung function by serial radiologic studies

37. Which of the following should be assessed to determine the benefit of long-acting β agonists in an asthmatic patient?
    1. Nocturnal symptoms
    2. Number of exacerbations
    3. Medication delivery device choice
    4. Days of absence from work related to symptoms
        a. 1 and 2 only
        b. 2 and 3 only
        c. 1, 2, and 3 only
        d. 1, 2, and 4 only

38. To manage severe asthma and avoid respiratory failure, intubation, and mechanical ventilation, which of the following methods of administration of inhaled adrenergic bronchodilation is recommended by the NAEPP EPR 3 guidelines?
    a. Small-volume nebulizer every 10 minutes × 5 times
    b. Small-volume nebulizer every 60 minutes × 3 times
    c. MDI, 12 to 20 puffs every 4 hours
    d. Continuous nebulizer, 10 to 15 mg/hr

39. Children being treated for asthma should use only which of the following in conjunction with a corticosteroid?
    a. Short-acting agonist
    b. Long-acting agonist
    c. α_1 Stimulator
    d. Catecholamine

40. The extended-release form of albuterol, VoSpire ER, is delivered in which of the following ways?
    a. Tablet
    b. pressurized MDI (pMDI)
    c. Breath-actuated MDI
    d. Liquid

CASE STUDY 1

A 12-year-old patient suffers from moderate asthma. He is receiving a regimen of cromolyn sodium and corticosteroid.

1. What would be the best choice of sympathomimetic bronchodilator to accompany this therapy?

2. What is the one condition in which the sympathomimetic bronchodilator you chose in question 1 would be likely to cause your patient problems?

CASE STUDY 2

You are an asthma educator working in a doctor's office. Candace is 27-year-old woman who has been diagnosed with asthma. She is ordered to receive a β_2 agonist by pMDI. You and the doctor are meeting with her to review her medications and answer any questions Candace may have at this time. After some discussion, the doctor leaves, but Candace would like the educator to answer more of her questions concerning her drugs.

1. Candace would like to know why she has to take this drug by inhalation instead of taking it by tablet or syrup.

2. Candace says she knows the drug helps her airways "open up," but asks whether there is any other way she could see whether her drug is working.

3. Candace would also like to know whether this drug has side effects.

4. Candace is concerned about the drug's effect on her heart. What can the educator tell her to do to monitor for this effect, and when should she be concerned about her heart rate?

5. Candace asks: "What if the β_2 agonist doesn't control my asthma? Is there another medication that I can take?"

7 Anticholinergic (Parasympatholytic) Bronchodilators

CHAPTER OUTLINE

Key Terms and Definitions
Clinical Indications for use
Specific Anticholinergic (Parasympatholytic) Agents
Clinical Pharmacology
Mode of Action
Clinical Application
Respiratory Care Assessment of Anticholinergic Bronchodilator Therapy
National Board of Respiratory Care (NBRC) Testing Questions
Case Studies 1 and 2

CHAPTER OBJECTIVES

After answering the following questions, the reader should be able to:

1. Define terms that pertain to anticholinergic bronchodilators
2. Differentiate between *parasympathomimetic* and *parasympatholytic*
3. Differentiate between *cholinergic* and *anticholinergic*
4. Differentiate between *muscarinic* and *antimuscarinic*
5. List all available anticholinergic agents used in respiratory therapy
6. Discuss the indication for anticholinergic agents
7. Explain the mode of action for anticholinergic agents
8. Identify the route of administration available for anticholinergic agents
9. Discuss adverse effects for anticholinergic agents
10. Discuss the clinical application for anticholinergic agents

KEY TERMS AND DEFINITIONS

Complete the following questions by writing the answer in the space provided.

1. What is the term used to describe an agent that blocks parasympathetic nervous fibers?

2. What is the term used to describe an agent that produces the effect of acetylcholine?

3. What is the term used to describe an agent that blocks parasympathetic nervous fibers, which allow relaxation of smooth muscle in the airway?

4. Which word has the same meaning as *cholinergic*, producing the effect of acetylcholine or an agent that mimics acetylcholine?

5. Which word has the same meaning as *anticholinergic*: blocking the effect of acetylcholine at the cholinergic site?

6. What is the term used to describe an agent that produces effects similar to those of the parasympathetic nervous system?

CLINICAL INDICATIONS FOR USE

Complete the following questions by writing the correct term in the blank provided.

7. List six anticholinergic bronchodilators that are indicated as a bronchodilator for maintenance and treatment in chronic obstructive pulmonary disease (COPD), including chronic bronchitis and emphysema (give generic and trade names).

Generic   **Trade**

a. _____   _____

b. _____   _____

c. _____   _____

d. _____   _____

e. _____   _____

f. _____   _____

8. What two types of medications are combined and indicated for use in patients needing regular treatment for COPD and who require additional bronchodilation for relief of airflow obstruction?

9. What two medications make up Combivent?

a. _____

b. _____

10. What is the trade name for the combination of umeclidinium and vilanterol?

11. What can Tiotropiam bromide be delivered?

12. What is the indication for use of Stiolto Respimat? Stiolto Respimat is a combination of what two medications?

13. You are taking care of a patient with severe asthma who has bronchoconstriction and is not responding well to β-agonist therapy. What medication can you suggest be delivered to this patient?

SPECIFIC ANTICHOLINERGIC (PARASYMPATHOLYTIC) AGENTS

Complete the following questions by writing in the blank provided.

14. List the brand names for the following.

a. Tiotropium bromide: _____

b. Ipratropium bromide: _____

c. Ipratropium bromide and albuterol (soft mist inhaler [SMI]): _____

d. Glycopyrrolate bromide and formoterol: _____

e. Aclidinium bromide: _____

f. Umeclidinium bromide: _____

g. Aclidinium Bromide and formoterol: _____

Match the administration method to the correct drug. (Some may require more than one answer.)

15. _____ MDI

16. _____ SMI

17. _____ SVN

18. _____ DPI

19. _____ VMN

a. Atrovent
b. Anoro Ellipta
c. Duaklir Pressair
d. Spiriva
e. Incruse Ellipta
f. Tudorza Pressair
g. Combivent Respimat
h. Stiolto Respimat
i. Yupelri
j. Bevespi Aerosphere
k. Lonhala Magnair

20. Complete the following table for inhaled anticholinergic bronchodilator agents.

Drug	Brand Name	Adult Dosage	Time Course (Onset, Peak, Duration)
Ipratropium bromide			*Onset:* *Peak:* *Duration:*
Ipratropium bromide and albuterol			*Onset:* *Peak:* *Duration:*
Aclidinium bromide			*Onset:* *Peak:* *Duration:*
Aclidinium bromide and formoterol			*Onset:* *Peak:* *Duration:*
Glycopyrrolate bromide			*Onset:* *Peak:* *Duration:*
Glycopyrrolate bromide and formoterol			*Onset:* *Peak:* *Duration:*
Revefenacin			*Onset:* *Peak:* *Duration:*
Tiotropium bromide			*Onset:* *Peak:* *Duration:*
Tiotropium bromide and olodaterol			*Onset:* *Peak:* *Duration:*
Umeclidinium bromide			*Onset:* *Peak:* *Duration:*
Umeclidinium bromide and vilanterol			*Onset:* *Peak:* *Duration:*

Chapter **7** Anticholinergic (Parasympatholytic) Bronchodilators

21. Explain how the clinical effect for ipratropium differs from that for albuterol.

22. Explain the receptor selectivity of tiotropium bromide. How does this explain once-a-day dosing?

23. Your patient has recently been prescribed umeclidinium bromide by his primary care physician and needs an explanation of how it works. What would you tell him?

24. What pharmacologic effects do ipratropium and tiotropium have on the respiratory and cardiac systems?

CLINICAL PHARMACOLOGY

25. Your patient has just received an inappropriately high dose of atropine. Explain the pharmacologic effects you would expect to see during a physical assessment.

MODE OF ACTION

26. Parasympathetic neurons from what cranial nerve enter the lung at the hila and travel along the airways?

27. Explain why the administration of an anticholinergic can cause significant bronchodilation.

Complete the following questions by writing the correct term in the blank provided.

28. Explain why methacholine is used in bronchial provocation testing.

29. Your patient is an 8-year-old female patient with persistent asthma not currently controlled with long-acting β-agonist and inhaled corticosteroid therapy. Which of the anticholinergics may help this patient?

30. When sensory C-fiber nerves are stimulated, what clinical manifestation may the patient present with?

68

31. List the two most common side effects seen with the anticholinergic aerosol ipratropium.

a. _____

b. _____

The following questions concern delivery of a quaternary ammonium antimuscarinic bronchodilator, such as ipratropium bromide.

CLINICAL APPLICATION

32. Complete the following table by comparing the general clinical effects of anticholinergic and β-adrenergic bronchodilators.

	Anticholinergic	β Agonist
a. Onset		
b. Time to peak effect		
c. Duration		
d. Fall in arterial partial pressure of oxygen (Pao_2)		
e. Site of action		

33. Where in the airway do anticholinergic bronchodilators seem to have their greatest effect?

34. Besides improving lung function in COPD and controlling symptoms, tiotropium may also be useful for controlling _____ _____ symptoms and deterioration of flow rates at nighttime.

35. Anticholinergics may be useful in patients with acute severe episodes of asthma not responding to _____.

36. Anticholinergics act primarily on the _____ airways; β agonists act primarily on the _____ airways.

37. True or False: Because albuterol peaks sooner and terminates sooner, and ipratropium peaks slowly and lasts longer, they complement each other.

38. Combined which two medication therapies may give additive bronchodilating results in COPD and in severe, acute asthma?

39. True or False: An anticholinergic bronchodilator, because of its action on central large airways, should be given before a β agonist.

40. Long-term agents that help reduce the progression of COPD and improve lung function have been termed *triple therapy*. Name the three agents that fall into this category.

a. _____

b. _____

c. _____

RESPIRATORY CARE ASSESSMENT OF ANTICHOLINERGIC BRONCHODILATOR THERAPY

41. List four respiratory care assessments you should perform before the delivery of anticholinergic bronchodilator therapy.

   a. _____

   b. _____

   c. _____

   d. _____

42. List two respiratory care assessments you should perform during the delivery of anticholinergic bronchodilator therapy.

   a. _____

   b. _____

43. List five respiratory care assessments you should perform after the delivery of and for long-term use of anticholinergic bronchodilator therapy.

   a. _____

   b. _____

   c. _____

   d. _____

   e. _____

NATIONAL BOARD OF RESPIRATORY CARE (NBRC) TESTING QUESTIONS

1. An agent that blocks parasympathetic nervous fibers, which allow relaxation of airway smooth muscle, is called:
   a. A parasympathomimetic
   b. An anticholinergic
   c. A muscarinic
   d. A cholinergic

2. A physician has written an order to give a patient Combivent HFA; the order provides no other information. How many puffs and how often should the patient receive this treatment?
   a. Two puffs, qid
   b. Two puffs, qd
   c. Two puffs, bid
   d. Two puffs, q4h

3. A patient calls the pulmonary rehabilitation department and tells the therapist that she has been taking Incruse Ellipta twice per day for the past 2 days. The respiratory therapist should tell the patient to:
   a. Continue on this routine
   b. Increase the treatment to three times per day
   c. Take the medication once per day
   d. Increase the treatment to four times per day

4. The total dose of Atrovent HFA in one puff is:
   a. 17 µg
   b. 34 µg
   c. 39 µg
   d. 100 µg

5. A drug with cholinergic effects would result in which of the following?
   1. Urination
   2. Salivation
   3. Secretion of mucus
   4. Increased heart rate
      a. 1 only
      b. 2 and 4 only
      c. 2, 3, and 4 only
      d. 1, 2, and 3 only

6. A parasympathomimetic agent that intensifies the level of bronchial tone to the point of bronchial constriction and is used in bronchial provocation testing is:
   a. Atropine
   b. Ipratropium
   c. Methacholine
   d. Tiotropium

7. Which of the following could be assessed to determine the effectiveness of tiotropium bromide?
   1. Keep a count of the number of exacerbations
   2. Keep a count of the number of unscheduled clinic visits
   3. Keep a count of the amount of sputum expectorated during exacerbations
   4. Keep a count of the number of hospitalizations
      a. 1 and 2 only
      b. 2 and 3 only
      c. 1, 2, and 4 only
      d. 2, 3, and 4 only

8. Which of the following describes quaternary ammonium compounds?
   a. They cross the blood–brain barrier.
   b. They are easily absorbed.
   c. They do not cause CNS changes.
   d. They are distributed throughout the body.

9. Anoro Ellipta is a combination of which two medications?
   a. Albuterol and umeclidinium bromide
   b. Vilanterol and umeclidinium bromide
   c. Vilanterol and ipratropium bromide
   d. Albuterol and tiotropium bromide

10. If ipratropium is delivered as an aerosol nebulizer treatment with a mask, what precautions should be taken?
    a. Pinch the nose of the patient.
    b. Stand outside the room.
    c. Caution the patient not to swallow.
    d. Protect the patient's eyes.

CASE STUDY 1

Jane has a 100 pack-year smoking history. She suffers from a combination of emphysema and chronic bronchitis. Lately, she has been increasingly more short of breath than usual, and her dyspnea is accompanied by some expiratory wheezing.

1. What do you think she will respond to better: sympathomimetic bronchodilators or anticholinergic bronchodilators?

2. If you choose combination therapy, such as ipratropium and albuterol, is it better to give each drug separately or as combined therapy?

CASE STUDY 2

A 74-year-old man with a history of COPD has been admitted to the hospital. The patient has been ordered to receive ipratropium.

1. Besides explaining to the patient why he has been prescribed this medication treatment, what would be important to tell the patient concerning a hazard of this medication?

2. The patient asks what the best way would be to administer the medication. What do you tell him?

After trying this technique, the patient requests that he would rather use an SVN because of his familiarity with this method.

3. How should the equipment be set up to avoid drug exposure to the eye?

The patient feels that the mouthpiece will be uncomfortable and requests the use of a mask.

4. What precautions should be taken by the patient to avoid eye contact with the drug?

Several days later, the patient is being discharged from the hospital. The patient has an order to continue ipratropium at home.

5. What aerosol inhalation technique would be best for this patient?

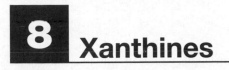

Xanthines

CHAPTER OUTLINE

Clinical Indications for Use of Xanthines
Specific Xanthine Agents
General Pharmacologic Properties
Titrating Theophylline Doses
Respiratory Care Assessment of Xanthines
National Board of Respiratory Care (NBRC) Testing Questions
Case Studies 1 and 2

CHAPTER OBJECTIVES

After answering the following questions, the reader should be able to:

1. Define *xanthine*
2. List all available xanthines used in respiratory therapy
3. Differentiate between the clinical indications of xanthines
4. Differentiate between the uses of xanthines
5. Discuss the proposed theories of activity for xanthines
6. Discuss adverse effects and toxicity of xanthines
7. Be able to assess xanthine therapy clinically

CLINICAL INDICATIONS FOR USE OF XANTHINES

Complete the following questions by writing the answer in the space provided, or by providing a brief answer.

1. List three indications for the use of xanthines.

   a. _____

   b. _____

   c. _____

2. Using the Global Initiative for Chronic Obstructive Lung Disease (GOLD) guidelines, explain when theophylline could be used as a treatment of chronic obstructive pulmonary disease (COPD). Are there any potential problems with its administration?

3. Explain the use of caffeine citrate in premature infants.

73

4. What benefit does caffeine citrate have over theophylline when treating premature infants for apnea of prematurity?

5. When prescribing theophylline, what must be considered in relation to the metabolism rates of individual patients?

SPECIFIC XANTHINE AGENTS

Complete the following questions by writing the correct term in the space provided.

6. List at least three available formulations of theophylline.

GENERAL PHARMACOLOGIC PROPERTIES

7. What are the three proposed mechanisms of action by which xanthines reverse airway obstruction?

    a. _____

    b. _____

    c. _____

TITRATING THEOPHYLLINE DOSES

8. Given the following levels of serum theophylline, indicate the effect each level could have on the body.

Micrograms (mcg)/Milliliter (mL)	Effect
a. < 5	
b. 10-20	
c. > 20	
d. > 30	
e. 40-45	

9. List six central nervous system (CNS) adverse reactions seen with theophylline treatment.

    a. _____

    b. _____

    c. _____

    d. _____

    e. _____

    f. _____

10. After administering an immediate-release form of theophylline when should serum blood levels should be obtained?

11. After administering a sustained-release form of theophylline when should serum blood levels should be measured?

12. Match the adverse reactions seen with theophylline with the organ system.

1. _____ Diuresis   a. CNS

2. _____ Tachypnea   b. Gastrointestinal

3. _____ Nausea   c. Respiratory

4. _____ Anxiety   d. Cardiovascular

5. _____ Palpitations   e. Renal

6. _____ Vomiting

7. _____ Headache

13. What precautions should you take when administering theophylline to patients with cystic fibrosis?

14. Where is Theophylline metabolized? Where is Theophylline excreted.

RESPIRATORY CARE ASSESSMENT OF XANTHINES

Identify each of the following statements as either true or false.

15. Describe a clinical situation in which Theophylline can be used for maintenance therapy in COPD?

16. List three nonbronchodilating effects of theophylline.

a. _____

b. _____

c. _____

NATIONAL BOARD OF RESPIRATORY CARE (NBRC) TESTING QUESTIONS

1. Theophylline is chemically referred to as one of which of the following drugs?
   a. β Blockers
   b. Anticholinergics
   c. Xanthines
   d. Aminophylline agonists

2. Which of the following physiologic effects are found in xanthines?
   1. Improvement in diaphragm muscle endurance
   2. Cardiac muscle suppression
   3. Diaphragm strengthening
   4. Diuresis
      a. 1 and 3 only
      b. 2 and 4 only
      c. 1, 3, and 4 only
      d. 1, 2, and 4 only

3. Compared with the β agonists, theophylline has what degree of bronchodilating *effect*?
   a. Weaker
   b. Comparable
   c. Stronger
   d. Much stronger

4. In the management of asthma, the therapeutic range for serum theophylline is which of the following?
   a. 2 to 12 mcg/mL
   b. 5 to 15 mcg/mL
   c. 20 to 30 mcg/mL
   d. More than 30 mcg/mL

5. Cardiovascular side effects associated with theophylline use include which of the following?
   1. Hypertension
   2. Ventricular arrhythmias
   3. Supraventricular tachycardia
   4. Palpitations
      a. 1 and 2 only
      b. 2 and 3 only
      c. 1, 3, and 4 only
      d. 2, 3, and 4 only

6. Theophylline may be used to treat which of the following?
   1. Pneumonia
   2. Apnea of prematurity
   3. COPD
   4. Asthma
      a. 1 and 4 only
      b. 2 and 3 only
      c. 2, 3, and 4 only
      d. 1, 2, and 4 only

7. Which of the following conditions can decrease the blood levels of theophylline?
   a. Cirrhosis
   b. Cigarette smoking
   c. Congestive heart failure
   d. Renal failure

8. Methylxanthines are considered first-line agents in the treatment of:
   a. Congestive heart failure
   b. Asthma
   c. COPD
   d. Apnea of prematurity

9. In which of the following formulations is theophylline available?
   1. Aerosol
   2. Intravenous
   3. Oral
   4. Rectal suppository
      a. 1 and 2 only
      b. 2 and 3 only
      c. 2, 3, and 4 only
      d. 1, 2, and 4 only

10. What does GOLD recommend for a therapeutic serum level of theophylline when treating COPD patients?
    a. 0 to 5 mcg/mL
    b. 5 to 10 mcg/mL
    c. 10 to 12 mcg/mL
    d. 10 to 20 mcg/mL

11. A serum blood theophylline level of 25 μg/mL has been determined for an adult patient in the emergency department. Which of the following effects may be seen with this serum level?
    a. No effects
    b. Cardiac arrhythmias
    c. Nausea and vomiting
    d. Seizures

12. A loading dose of _____ mg/kg of caffeine has been found effective in treating apnea of prematurity.
    a. 0.5
    b. 5
    c. 10
    d. 20

13. It is suggested that giving a patient with COPD theophylline has nonbronchodilating effects. These effects would include:
    1. Ventilatory drive stimulation
    2. Reduced bronchial secretions
    3. Enhanced respiratory muscle function
    4. Anti-inflammatory effects
        a. 2 and 4 only
        b. 1 and 3 only
        c. 1, 3, and 4 only
        d. 2, 3, and 4 only

14. Which of the following factors increase the blood serum levels of theophylline?
    1. Alcohol
    2. Calcium channel blockers
    3. Albuterol
    4. Corticosteroids
        a. 1 and 3 only
        b. 2 and 3 only
        c. 1, 2, and 4 only
        d. 2, 3, and 4 only

15. Theophylline is contraindicated in which of the following?
    a. Glaucoma
    b. Active peptic ulcer
    c. Diabetes
    d. Acute kidney disease

16. Why is theophylline recommended only as an alternative to inhaled bronchodilators in the treatment of COPD?
    a. It produces excessive secretions.
    b. Acute gastritis is produced.
    c. It reduces forced expiratory volume at 1 second (FEV_1) over long-term administration.
    d. It has potential toxicity because of the narrow therapeutic margin.

17. When administering caffeine, which of the following has the greatest intensity of effects?
    a. Cardiac stimulation
    b. Skeletal muscle stimulation
    c. Diuresis
    d. Smooth muscle relaxation

18. On checking the medical chart of a patient with COPD, you observe the patient has received an immediate-release form of theophylline as a loading dose at 1300. What time should you go back to monitor serum theophylline levels on this patient?
    a. 1430
    b. 1700
    c. 1830
    d. 2200

19. A patient receives a sustained-release form of theophylline in the morning. When should a serum theophylline level be obtained?
    a. 5 to 9 hours later
    b. 13 to 15 hours later
    c. 1 to 2 hours later
    d. 24 hours later

20. How is theophylline removed from the body?
    a. Metabolized by the liver
    b. Removed by the kidney
    c. Removed by the gastrointestinal tract
    d. Metabolized by the kidney

CASE STUDY 1

Joe has been recently diagnosed with COPD. He is 57, has worked in the coal mines since he was 17, and suffers from severe dyspnea. Joe's physician prescribed oxygen for home use at 2 L/min, β agonists, and corticosteroids. Joe has not responded as his physician had hoped. (Joe has had no change in his FEV_1.) Joe's physician has decided to initiate sustained-release theophylline and asks you to calculate the appropriate dose for Joe, who weighs 75 kg and is 6 feet tall.

1. What dose should Joe begin with?

The following day, Joe calls his physician and states that he feels no improvement. The doctor suggests to Joe that he will increase Joe's dose, but he will need to check Joe's theophylline level first.

2. When is the best time to do this?

Joe's serum level comes back as 5 mcg/mL. Joe still feels no change or improvement since starting the medication.

3. What should be recommended?

4. Are there any other medications that can be added to his daily regimen?

Baby Ladarius is a 1500-g, 32-week gestational age newborn who has been in neonatal intensive care for 2 days for laboratory workup and monitoring for irregular breathing and desaturation. Over the last 12 hours, baby Ladarius has had increased episodes of apnea for 30 seconds and brady-cardia accompanied by cyanosis. Baby Ladarius requires tactile stimulation to resume breathing. On stimulation, he resumes breathing, and his heart rate and saturation normalize. The respiratory therapist suggests that baby Ladarius has apnea of prematurity, and after consultation with the doctor, the doctor agrees.

1. Based on baby Ladarius's symptoms, what would be considered the first-line medication of choice?

2. The nurse suggests that baby Ladarius receives theophylline to treat his apnea. What do you think about this suggestion?

3. The nurse still believes that theophylline would be better for baby Ladarius because of the nurse's experience with this drug. What else could you tell her to convince her of your suggestion?

4. Okay. The nurse is convinced. What would be the appropriate loading dose of this medication?

5. Twenty-four hours later, baby Ladarius is still having episodes of apnea and bradycardia. What recommendation would you suggest?

CHAPTER OUTLINE

CHAPTER OBJECTIVES

After answering the following questions, the reader should be able to:

1. Define terms that pertain to mucus-controlling drug therapy
2. Interpret the physiology and mechanisms of mucus secretion and clearance
3. Name the types of mucoactive medications and their presumed modes of action
4. Describe the medications approved for the therapy of mucus clearance disorders and their approved indications
5. Identify the contraindications to the use of mucoactive medications
6. Explain the interaction between airway clearance devices or physical therapy and mucoactive medications

KEY TERMS AND DEFINITIONS

Match the following definitions with their terms.

1. _____ Macromolecular description of pseudoplastic material having both viscosity and elasticity.

2. _____ Medication that increases cough or ciliary clearance of respiratory secretions.

3. _____ The study of deformation and flow of matter in response to an applied stress.

4. _____ Medication meant to increase the volume or hydration of airway secretions.

a. Elasticity
b. Expectorant
c. Gel
d. Mucin
e. Mucoactive agent
f. Mucokinetic agent
g. Mucolytic agent
h. Mucoregulatory agent
i. Mucospissic
j. Mucus
k. Rheology

5. _____ The principal constituent of mucus.

6. _____ Resistance of liquid to sheer forces or energy loss with applied stress.

7. _____ Medication that degrades polymers in secretions.

8. _____ Secretion, from surface goblet cells and submucosal glands, composed of water, proteins, and glycosylated mucins.

9. _____ Term connoting any medication or drug that has an effect on mucus secretion.

10. _____ Expectorated secretions that contain respiratory tract, oropharyngeal, and nasopharyngeal secretions, as well as bacteria and products of inflammation, including polymeric DNA and actin.

11. _____ A drug that reduces the volume of airway mucus secretion and appears to be especially effective in hypersecretory states.

12. _____ Rheologic property characteristic of solids.

13. _____ A medication that increases the viscosity of secretions and may be effective in the therapy of bronchorrhea.

14. _____ Protein that gives mucus its physical/chemical properties, such as viscoelasticity.

15. _____ Referred to as the periciliary layer.

16. _____ Sugar that is the individual carbohydrate unit of glycoprotein.

17. _____ Purulent material in the airways.

l. Sputum
m. Viscosity
n. Glycoprotein
o. Sol
p. Oligosaccharide
q. Phlegm

DRUG CONTROL OF MUCUS: A PERSPECTIVE

18. When should mucoactive therapy be considered?

19. List five factors of mucus that are beneficial regardless of its location.

    a. _____

    b. _____

    c. _____

    d. _____

    e. _____

20. For the mucoactive agents listed, provide the following information:

Drug	Brand Name	Use	Adult Dose
N-acetylcysteine-L-cysteine (NAC)			
Dornase alfa			
Aqueous water, saline (0.9%)	N/A		
Hyperosmolar saline 7%			
Dry powder mannitol			
3% hyperosmolar saline	N/A		

21. What are the two airway mucus layers called? Briefly describe each.

    a. _____

    b. _____

22. Explain the difference between mucus and sputum.

23. Complete the following table concerning the effects of various drug groups on mucociliary clearance.

Drug Group	Ciliary Beat	Mucus Production
α-Adrenergic agents		
Cholinergic agents		
Methylxanthines		
Corticosteroids		
Anticholinergics		

NATURE OF MUCUS SECRETIONS

24. List seven factors that can slow mucociliary transport.

    a. _____

    b. _____

    c. _____

    d. _____

    e. _____

    f. _____

    g. _____

25. What is considered the most important predisposing factor to airway irritation and mucus hypersecretion, but other factors can include viral infections, pollutants, and genetic predisposition in patients with chronic bronchitis?

26. Briefly describe each of the following disease states and give a reason each may require mucus-controlling drug therapy.
    a. Chronic bronchitis:
    b. Asthma:
    c. Bronchorrhea:
    d. Plastic bronchitis:
    e. Cystic fibrosis (CF):

27. What is the main component of the sectetions in the airways of patients with Cystic fibrosis?

28. Why is it so difficult for a person with purulent sputum to cough it up?

MUCOACTIVE AGENTS

29. Discuss two therapeutic options, besides using mucoactive agents, for controlling mucus hypersecretion.

    a. _____

    b. _____

30. NAC works by disrupting _____ _____ and is more effective in alkaline pH environments.

31. When administering NAC by aerosol how can the incidence of bronchospasm can be reduced?

32. List a nonrespiratory indication for the use of NAC.

33. Why is dornase alfa not prescribed for patients with bronchiectasis and chronic obstructive pulmonary disease (COPD)?

34. List three indications for the use of dornase alfa:

    a. _____

    b. _____

    c. _____

35. What nebulizers and compressors have been approved for delivery of dornase alfa?

    a. _____

    b. _____

    c. _____

36. How would you evaluate the effectiveness of dornase alfa in a patient with CF?

Mucolytics and Expectorants

37. Guaifenesin has been approved by the U.S. Food and Drug Administration (FDA) as a bilayer extended-release tablet and as an expectorant called _____.

Mucokinetic agents

38. What disease would benefit from increased expiratory airflow with the use of α agonists?

39. Your patient has been diagnosed with tracheomalacia. She has taken α agonists in the past, but her physician suggested to stop. Can you explain to her why?

MUCOREGULATORY MEDICATIONS

40. The long-term use of a mucoregulatory medication such as ipratropium is associated with a reduction in the volume of mucus secretion in patients with what diagnosis?

OTHER MUCOACTIVE AGENTS

41. In what disease would antiproteases be helpful in restoring the bacteria-killing capacity of neutrophils?

42. Why is hyperosmolar saline (hypertonic saline) thought to improve mucociliary transport?

43. A patient with CF has been prescribed hyperosmolar therapy using a 7% hypertonic saline solution administered twice daily (bid). What recommended delivery device should be used for this therapy?

GENE THERAPY

44. What is necessary for gene therapy to be effective?

45. What is an example of viral vector?

USING MUCOACTIVE THERAPY WITH PHYSICAL THERAPY AND AIRWAY CLEARANCE DEVICES

46. What is the difference between a directed cough and a huff cough?

47. True or False: Conventional chest physical therapy (CPT) incorporating postural drainage results in significantly greater expectoration than no treatment in patients with CF.

48. True or False: The insufflation-exsufflation device inflates the lungs with positive pressure followed by a negative pressure to simulate a cough.

49. True or False: The active cycle of breathing techniques uses relaxed diaphragmatic breathing and the insufflation-exsufflation device.

50. True or False: Autogenic drainage incorporates staged breathing, starting with small tidal breaths from expiratory reserve volume (ERV), repeated until secretions "collect" in the central airways. It is recommended for patients more than 8 years of age.

51. True or False: Exercise, if tolerated, should be substituted for other bronchial hygiene regimens.

52. With what airway clearance device does the patient breathe through a mouthpiece that delivers high-flow minibursts at rates exceeding 200 cycles/min?

53. Which airway clearance device provides pressure pulses that fill a vest and vibrate the chest wall at variable frequencies applied during the entire respiratory cycle?

54. *Match the descriptions to the appropriate airway clearance method.*

1. _____ Mr. Cilia is a 69-year-old patient with COPD. He uses this positive airway pressure (PAP) technique as an effective alternative to CPT in expanding the lungs and mobilizing secretions.

2. _____ Randolph is a 32-year-old patient with CF and uses this device when he is traveling. This device combines positive expiratory pressure (PEP) with high-frequency oscillations at the airway opening.

3. _____ Robin is a 29-year-old who has CF. She is a salesperson for a pharmaceutical company, travels extensively, and is very motivated. The airway clearance technique she uses incorporates staged breathing starting with small tidal breaths from ERV, repeated until secretions "collect" in the central airways. It is recommended for patients more than 8 years of age.

4. _____ Ronald is an 18-year-old student with CF, and he is attending his first year of college away from home. Because he is independent and must perform his own therapy, the airway clearance device he uses provides pressure pulses that fill a vest and vibrate the chest wall at variable frequencies applied during the entire respiratory cycle. He uses it for 20-30 minutes per treatment and takes his nebulized medication at the same time.

5. _____ Alfred is a 22-year-old man with CF. He does not tolerate or like any other device except this one, which provides breaths through a mouthpiece and delivers high-flow minibursts at rates exceeding 200 cycles/min.

6. _____ Mary is a 44-year-old woman with cerebral palsy. She has poor coughing and limited expiratory airflow. When in the hospital, she uses this device, which can generate high-frequency oscillations at the airway opening or on the chest wall.

7. _____ Lauren is 18 years old and has cerebral palsy and severe scoliosis. This device inflates her lungs with positive pressure, followed by negative pressure to simulate a cough.

8. _____ Jasmin has just taken a job as a traveling respiratory therapist. Jasmin has CF and believes it would be best to use a technique that allows her not to take equipment with her. Her CF clinic taught her this airway clearance technique. It is a combination of breathing control (relaxed diaphragmatic breathing), thoracic expansion control (deep breaths), and a forced expiration technique from progressively increasing lung volumes.

a. Chest wall oscillation: The Vest
b. FLUTTER mucus clearance device
c. Autogenic drainage
d. Active cycle of breathing technique
e. An insufflation-exsufflation device
f. Pursed-lip breathing
g. Intrapulmonary percussive ventilation

1. A mucokinetic medication is one that:
   a. Increases ciliary clearance of respiratory mucus secretions
   b. Increases the volume or hydration of airway secretions
   c. Degrades polymers in secretions
   d. Increases ciliary activity

2. Pulmozyme is used primarily for:
   a. Chronic bronchitis
   b. Sputum induction
   c. CF
   d. Bronchitis

3. How would you evaluate the effectiveness of dornase alfa in the patient with CF?
   1. Reduction in intravenous (IV) antibiotic use
   2. Reduced need for hospitalizations
   3. Stability of lung function
   4. Reduced number and severity of infectious exacerbations
      a. 1 and 2 only
      b. 3 and 4 only
      c. 1, 3, and 4 only
      d. 1, 2, 3, and 4

4. Which of the following cells or glands is most likely responsible for the majority of mucus secretion?
   a. Ciliated epithelial cells
   b. Goblet cells
   c. Clara cells
   d. Submucosal glands

5. Which of the following forces severely reduces the ability to clear secretions by coughing?
   a. Viscosity
   b. Adhesion
   c. Elasticity
   d. Spinnability

6. Which of the following drugs increases ciliary beat?
   1. α Adrenergics
   2. Cholinergics
   3. Methylxanthines
   4. Corticosteroids
      a. 2 and 4 only
      b. 1 and 3 only
      c. 1, 2, and 3 only
      d. 1, 2, 3, and 4

7. Which of the following is considered the most important predisposing factor to airway irritation and mucus hyper-secretion with chronic bronchitis?
   a. Viral infections
   b. Tobacco smoke
   c. Pollutants
   d. Genetic predisposition

8. CF is associated with chronic airway infection, most often caused by:
   a. *Pseudomonas aeruginosa*
   b. *Staphylococcus aureus*
   c. *Streptococcus aureus*
   d. *Haemophilus influenzae*

9. Which of the following are therapeutic options for controlling mucus hypersecretion, other than using mucoactive agents?
    1. Remove causative factors, such as pollution, where possible.
    2. Treat infections.
    3. Optimize tracheobronchial clearance, including the use of bronchodilators.
    4. Incorporate bronchial hygiene measures, such as cough and postural drainage.
        a. 1 and 2 only
        b. 2 and 3 only
        c. 1, 3, and 4 only
        d. 1, 2, 3, and 4

10. Which of the following is considered to be a mucoactive agent?
    a. Dornase alfa
    b. Acetylcysteine
    c. Budesonide
    d. Sodium bicarbonate

11. When administering NAC by aerosol, it is important to include pretreatment with which of the following to reduce the incidence of bronchospasm?
    a. Short-acting β agonist
    b. Corticosteroid
    c. Cholinergic medication
    d. Expectorant

12. Opened vials of NAC should be:
    a. A purple color
    b. Stored in a refrigerator
    c. Stored in a lighted area that is room temperature
    d. Pink in color

13. Which of the following is suggested equipment for nebulization of dornase alfa?
    1. Hudson Updraft II
    2. Acorn II
    3. Pari LC Jet Plus
    4. Hamilton Fat Boy II
        a. 1 and 4 only
        b. 2 and 3 only
        c. 1, 2, and 3 only
        d. 2, 3, and 4 only

14. Common side effects with the use of dornase alfa include:
    1. Voice alteration
    2. Pharyngitis
    3. Thrush
    4. Laryngitis
        a. 1 and 3 only
        b. 2 and 4 only
        c. 1, 2, and 3 only
        d. 1, 2, and 4 only

15. NAC can be used to treat overdose of which of the following?
    a. Opiates
    b. Tylenol
    c. Motrin
    d. Valium

16. A patient with CF has been prescribed hyperosmolar therapy using a 7% hypertonic saline solution administered bid. What recommended delivery device should be used for this therapy?
    a. Hudson Updraft II
    b. Ultrasonic Nebulizer
    c. Pari LC Jet Plus
    d. Hamilton Fat Boy II

17. What percent hypertonic saline is recommended for use to induce a cough and improve mucociliary transport and lung function in CF?
    a. 7
    b. 5
    c. 3
    d. 0.9

18. Which of the following assessments is best for drug therapy for respiratory secretions to determine changes in the lung resulting from mucociliary clearance?
    a. FEV_1
    b. Change in lung function over time
    c. Vital capacity
    d. Peak flow rate

19. The surface of the trachea and bronchi includes primarily which of the following types of cells?
    1. Columnar epithelium
    2. Ciliated cells
    3. Goblet cells
    4. Pseudostratified cells
        a. 2 and 3 only
        b. 1 and 4 only
        c. 1, 3, and 4 only
        d. 2, 3, and 4 only

20. Which of the following is a reason that NAC should not be used as a mucoactive medication?
    a. The sulfur ingredient disrupts important mucins.
    b. It increases epithelial mucus and chloride secretion.
    c. It does not improve mucus clearance when given as an aerosol.
    d. It swells the mucus and causes reduced expectoration resulting from small airway blockage.

CASE STUDY

Johnny is a 6-year-old boy recently diagnosed with CF. Dr. Choo has just met with Johnny and his parents. They have come to your office for instruction and answers regarding the respiratory care Johnny will be receiving. Dr. Choo has ordered dornase alfa (Pulmozyme) and The Vest airway clearance system for Johnny. Johnny is to return for a follow-up visit in two weeks.

1. The parents want to know what equipment they will need to deliver the dornase alfa to Johnny and how often he should get it.

2. Because the equipment and medication are new to Johnny and his parents, what should you instruct them to do regarding Johnny's physical assessment so they feel more confident with this new therapy?

3. The parents know a child with CF who is 13 years old and does autogenic drainage and percussion and postural drainage, which do not require equipment. Can Johnny be taught this now and use this instead of The Vest?

4. Are any side effects associated with dornase alfa (Pulmozyme)?

5. Johnny has been using The Vest off and on for the past few months, but his parents forget how much pulse frequency to use. They believe it is somewhere about 5 Hz but are unsure. What should the respiratory therapist tell his parents?

6. What if Johnny doesn't tolerate or like The Vest? Can he switch to something else?

10 Surfactant Agents

CHAPTER OBJECTIVES

After answering the following questions, the reader should be able to:

1. Define key terms that pertain to surfactant agents
2. List all available exogenous surfactant agents used in respiratory therapy
3. Describe the mode of action for exogenous surfactant agents
4. Discuss the route of administration for exogenous surfactant agents
5. Recognize hazards and complications of exogenous surfactant therapy
6. Assess the use of surfactant therapy

KEY TERMS AND DEFINITIONS

Complete the following questions by writing the answer in the space provided.

1. What is the term used to describe a surface-active agent designed to lower surface tension?

2. What is the term used to describe the force caused by the attraction between like molecules, which occur at the liquid–gas interface, and that holds the liquid surface intact?

3. Explain why liquid molecules "draw in" on themselves and result in a spherical shape.

4. Laplace's Law describes and quantifies the relationship among:

    a. _____

    b. _____

    c. _____

5. Why is Laplace's Law different in the alveoli?

6. As Laplace's Law applies to the lung, the _____ the surface tension, the greater the compressing force inside the alveolus, which can lead to _____ of the alveolus.

IDENTIFICATION OF SURFACTANT PREPARATIONS

7. Fill in the following table of exogenous surfactant preparations currently used for the treatment of neonatal RDS.

Drug	Brand Name	Formulation and Initial Dose
Beractant		
Calfactant		
Poractant alfa		

EXOGENOUS SURFACTANTS

8. What is the key to the use of exogenous surfactant?

9. When is exogenous surfactant clinically indicated in the newborn infant?

10. What is the term used to describe surfactant treatment that is intended to help prevent respiratory distress syndrome (RDS) in very-low-birth-weight infants, and in higher-birth-weight infants who have evidence of immature lungs and who are at risk for developing RDS?

11. What term is used to describe the retroactive treatment for infants who have developed RDS?

Composition of Pulmonary Surfactant
Complete the following questions by writing the answer in the space provided.

12. What is the primary function of surfactant in the lung?

13. What component of the phospholipids in surfactant is primarily responsible for reduction of alveolar surface tension?

14. What is the major stimulus for surfactant secretion?

15. What is the estimated half-life of surfactant?

16. What is the term used for where surfactant lipids are synthesized and stored in type II alveolar cells in vesicles?

17. Based on the figure below, what change has occurred to the pressure–volume curve after administration of surfactant to the lung?

Exogenous surfactant

• High surface tension
• Low compliance
• Increased work of breathing

A

• Lower surface tension
• Increased compliance
• Decreased work of breathing

B

■ A: RDS (without surfactant)
□ B: After surfactant

V_T (mL)

Pressure (cm H_2O)

Types of Exogenous Surfactant Preparations
Complete the following questions by writing the answer in the space provided.

18. What type of surfactants are obtained from animals or humans by alveolar wash or from amniotic fluid?

19. Survanta and Infasurf come from _____ lungs, and Curosurf comes from _____ lungs.

SPECIFIC EXOGENOUS SURFACTANT PREPARATIONS

Complete the following questions by writing the answer in the space provided.

20. List two indications for the use of beractant (Survanta).

a. _____

b. _____

21. What protein is missing from Survanta? What effect could this have on the duration of effect?

22. Describe how you would warm Survanta prior to its use.

23. How is a dose of Survanta administered?

24. What is the recommended dose of Survanta?

25. List two indications for the use for calfactant (Infasurf).

    a. _____

    b. _____

26. How many repeat doses of Infasurf can be delivered?

27. How is a dose of Infasurf administered?

28. What is the recommended dose of Infasurf?

29. List two indications for the use of poractant alfa (Curosurf).

    a. _____

    b. _____

30. Describe how an infant is positioned during administration of Curosurf.

31. What is the recommended dose of Curosurf?

32. List three observations that would indicate that a newborn infant has responded well to administration of exogenous surfactant:

    a. _____

    b. _____

    c. _____

33. List three possible hazards of surfactant delivery.

    a. _____

    b. _____

    c. _____

NATIONAL BOARD OF RESPIRATORY CARE (NBRC) TESTING QUESTIONS

1. Surfactant accomplishes which of the following?
   a. Decreases lung compliance
   b. Lowers surface tension
   c. Forces pulmonary blood flow to perfuse nonventilated alveoli
   d. Improves mucociliary escalator

2. Which of the following happens as the surface tension of the liquid lining of the alveolus increases?
   a. More pulmonary blood flow perfuses the alveoli.
   b. It becomes more difficult for the alveolus to inflate.
   c. Airway resistance decreases.
   d. More type I cells are produced.

3. Which of the following cells is responsible for surfactant production?
   a. Type I
   b. Type II
   c. Type III
   d. Macrophage

4. Which term describes surfactant preparations from outside the patient's own body?
   a. Endogenous
   b. Exogenous
   c. Synthetic-type
   d. Detergent-type

5. Surfactant is composed of which of the following?
   a. Various amino acids
   b. 10% lipids and 90% proteins
   c. 50% lipids and 50% proteins
   d. 90% lipids and 10% proteins

6. How is exogenous surfactant administered?
   a. Aerosol route
   b. Direct instillation into the trachea
   c. Intravenously (IV)
   d. Parenteral route

7. Which of the following is Laplace's Law as it relates to the alveoli?
   a. 4 × surface tension/radius
   b. 4 × radius/surface tension
   c. 2 × radius/surface tension
   d. 2 × surface tension/radius

8. What would be the initial dose of Infasurf administered for prophylactic treatment of a newborn infant weighing 1 kg?
   a. 2.5 mL in four equally divided doses
   b. 3.0 mL in two equally divided doses
   c. 3.5 mL in four equally divided doses
   d. 4.0 mL in two equally divided doses

9. What is the reason that exogenously administered surfactant is successful in replacing surfactant in the lung after one or two doses?
   a. It is taken into the surfactant pool and recycled.
   b. Blood flow improves and allows more surfactant to be produced.
   c. It completely covers the inside of the alveoli surface.
   d. It improves compliance and increases oxygenation, and thus produces more surfactant.

10. Which of the following is primarily responsible for reduction of alveolar surface tension?
    a. Sphingomyelin
    b. Surfactant protein D
    c. Lecithin
    d. Surfactant protein A

11. The major stimulus for surfactant secretion is believed to be:
    a. Baroreceptors
    b. Chemoreceptors
    c. Pulmonary artery blood flow
    d. Lung inflation

12. Prophylactic Infasurf treatment is indicated for:
    a. Term infants with meconium aspiration syndrome (MAS)
    b. Infants less than 29 weeks of gestational age at risk for developing RDS
    c. Infants with group B streptococcus pneumonia (GBS)
    d. Infants more than 72 hours of age at risk for developing RDS

13. Two hours after administration of exogenous surfactant, an infant receiving mechanical ventilation shows an increase in exhaled tidal volume, from 4 to 8 mL/kg of body weight, with no change in pressure delivery. These findings would indicate:
    a. Reduced airway resistance
    b. Increased lung compliance
    c. Increased work of breathing
    d. The need to administer another dose of surfactant

14. An intubated infant just received a dose of Curosurf through a 5-French catheter. The infant is being hand ventilated with 90% oxygen. Suddenly, the infant's heart rate drops from 140 to 75 beats/min, Spo2 decreases from 89% to 70%, and work of breathing and retractions increase. The respiratory therapist should make which of the following recommendations:
    a. Extubate and manually ventilate the infant.
    b. Turn the infant so the opposite lung is dependent.
    c. Suction the ETT.
    d. Reconnect the infant to the ventilator.

15. The respiratory therapist reports to the physician that an infant has had a good response to administration of Curosurf, as indicated by:
    1. Increase in Pa_{O_2}
    2. Increase in Pa_{CO_2}
    3. Increase in lung compliance
        a. 1 only
        b. 2 and 3 only
        c. 1 and 3 only
        d. 1, 2, and 3

16. Natural surfactant is obtained from:
    1. Lungs of cows
    2. Lungs of pigs
    3. Lungs of horses
        a. 1 only
        b. 1 and 2 only
        c. 2 and 3 only
        d. 1, 2, and 3

17. Survanta administered as a rescue treatment for infants with evidence of RDS should occur:
    a. Within 8 hours of birth
    b. Immediately after birth
    c. Within 2 hours of birth
    d. Within 1 hour of birth

18. How much Survanta should be administered for prophylactic treatment of a newborn weighing 700 g?
    a. 2.8 mL
    b. 2.1 mL
    c. 4.0 mL
    d. 4.2 mL

19. A mechanically ventilated newborn infant is receiving Curosurf through an ETT. The respiratory therapist observes that the ETT has become obstructed during instillation, and the infant has desaturated and become bradycardic. Which of the following is recommended?
    a. Increase positive end expiratory pressure (PEEP)
    b. Increase fraction of inspired oxygen (FiO_2)
    c. Increase inspiratory time
    d. Manually ventilate

20. After administration of Infasurf, which of the following clinical changes would indicate improvement in lung mechanics?
    1. Increased compliance
    2. Reduced body temperature
    3. Decreased work of breathing
    4. Reduction in pulmonary secretions
       a. 1 and 3 only
       b. 1, 2, and 3 only
       c. 2, 3, and 4 only
       d. 1, 2, and 4 only

CASE STUDY 1

A male newborn infant with a gestational age of 26 weeks and birth weight of 900 g is in the neonatal intensive care unit (NICU). The 4-hour-old infant has been diagnosed with RDS and is intubated and has been receiving mechanical ventilation since birth. The decision has been made to administer Survanta. This baby fits the protocol's inclusion criteria, and you have been asked to talk to the parents about this decision.

1. How would you explain to the parents why exogenous surfactant is needed?

2. The parents would like to know how you will determine whether their child is getting better after administration of exogenous surfactant. What do you tell them?

After talking with you, the parents consent to the treatment. You return to the NICU and prepare to administer Survanta.

3. You notice that settling has occurred within the vial. How should it be mixed?

4. How much of the 8-mL vial will the infant require for the first dose if you are administering it through a side-port adaptor?

5. How would you position the baby for each dose?

6. You return to the parents and explain the procedure to them. They ask: "What will happen if he doesn't get better? Can he receive more surfactant?" What would you tell them?

A 25-week gestational age newborn weighing 600 g has been intubated with a 2.5-mm ETT and is receiving mechanical ventilation. Current ventilator settings are peak inspiratory pressure 20 cm H_2O, exhaled tidal volume 4 mL, inspiratory time 3 seconds, respiratory rate 40/min, positive end-expiratory pressure 4 cm H_2O, Fio_2 0.80. Physical assessment includes pulse 142/min, blood pressure 38/24 mm Hg, Spo_2 85%, temperature 99.6° F. A recent chest radiograph shows findings supportive of RDS. Based on the infant's current ventilatory support and chest x-ray finding, it is decided to administer Curosurf.

1. What is the recommended initial dose of Curosurf that should be administered?

2. What is the protocol for administration of Curosurf?

3. The infant has now received two doses of Curosurf. Over this period of time, the pressure-volume (PV) curve has changed from A to B, as imaged in the figure. Curve A represents when the infant was first mechanically ventilated, and curve B represents the PV curve after the second dose of Curosurf. What change in lung mechanics has occurred that is represented in PV curve B?

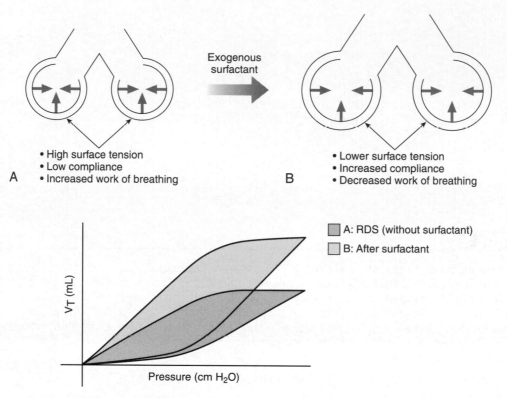

4. Based on the changes seen in curve B in the image in question #3, what are three potential complications that may develop?

    a. _____

    b. _____

    c. _____

11 Corticosteroids in Respiratory Care

CHAPTER OUTLINE

CHAPTER OBJECTIVES

After answering the following questions, the reader should be able to:

1. Define key terms that pertain to corticosteroids
2. Discuss the indications for inhaled corticosteroid use
3. List all available inhaled corticosteroids used in respiratory therapy
4. Differentiate among specific corticosteroid formulations
5. Describe the route of administration available for corticosteroids
6. Describe the mode of action for corticosteroids
7. Discuss the effect corticosteroids have on the white blood cell count
8. Discuss the effect corticosteroids have on β receptors
9. Differentiate between systemic and local side effects of corticosteroids
10. Discuss the use of corticosteroids in the treatment of asthma and chronic obstructive pulmonary disease
11. Be able to clinically assess corticosteroid use in patient care

KEY TERMS AND DEFINITIONS

Complete the following questions by writing the answer in the space provided.

1. What does the term steroid diabetes refer to?

2. Define endogenous.

3. What gamma globulin produced by cells in the respiratory tract?

4. What hormone-type substance, is an inflammatory mediator and part of the arachidonic acid cascade?

5. What response do glucocorticoids, or steroids produce in the body?

6. What are chemicals secreted by the adrenal cortex are called?

7. Define exogenous.

8. What are chemical mediators and when are they released?

CLINICAL INDICATION FOR USE OF INHALED CORTICOSTEROIDS

Complete the following questions by writing the answer in the space provided.

9. List two formulations in which inhaled corticosteroids are available.

   a. _____

   b. _____

10. At what level of care in asthma, as defined by the National Asthma Education and Prevention Program (NAEPP) Expert Panel Report 3 *Guidelines for the Diagnosis and Management of Asthma—Update on Selected Topics,* are corticosteroids clinically indicated?

11. In severe asthma, both inhaled corticosteroids are combined with what other type of corticosteroids?

12. List two clinical indications for intranasal aerosolized corticosteroids.

   a. _____

   b. _____

13. Match the following aerosolized corticosteroids for oral inhalation with their brand name.

Drug

1. _____ Mometasone furoate
2. _____ Beclomethasone dipropionate HFA
3. _____ Fluticasone propionate/salmeterol
4. _____ Ciclesonide
5. _____ Budesonide/formoterol fumarate HFA
6. _____ Fluticasone propionate
7. _____ Flunisolide furoate
8. _____ Budesonide
9. _____ Mometasone furoate/formoterol fumarate HFA
10. _____ Fluticasone furoate/vilanterol
11. _____ Fluticasone furoate/umeclidinium bromidevilanterol
12. _____ Budesonide/glycopyrrolate/formoterol

Brand Name

a. Arnuity Ellipta
b. QVAR RediHaler
c. Pulmicort Flexhaler, Pulmicort Respules
d. Asmanex HFA, Asmanex Twisthaler
e. Advair HFA, Advair Diskus, AirDuo Respiclick/Digihaler, Wixela Inhub
f. Symbicort
g. Flovent HFA, Flovent Diskus
h. Alvesco
i. Dulera
j. Breo Ellipta
k. Trelegy Elipta
l. Breztri Aerosphere

14. Match the following aerosolized corticosteroids for intranasal delivery with their brand name.

Drug	Brand Name
1. _____ Triamcinolone acetonide	a. Nasonex
2. _____ Olopatadine hydrochloride/mometasone furoate	b. Beconase AQ, Qnasl
3. _____ Fluticasone	c. Rhinocort, Rhinocort Allergy
4. _____ Budesonide	d. Flonase Allergy Relief
5. _____ Mometasone furoate	e. Nasacort Allergy 24 Hour
6. _____ Beclomethasone	f. Ryaltris
7. _____ Ciclesonide	g. Omnaris, Zetonna

PHYSIOLOGY OF CORTICOSTEROIDS

Identification and Source

15. What effect do glucocorticoids exert in the body?

16. List two side effects of glucocorticoids.

    a. _____

    b. _____

17. What is a primary reason for using aerosolized glucocorticoids versus systemic ones?

18. What can you do to help prevent acute severe episodes of asthma that may happen while withdrawing a patient from oral steroids?

NATURE OF THE INFLAMMATORY RESPONSE

19. Name two of the most common inflammatory lung diseases.

    a. _____

    b. _____

20. Give a description of each category of the triple response to inflammation.

    a. _____

    b. _____

    c. _____

INFLAMMATION IN THE AIRWAY

21. Evidence indicates that the early asthmatic response is caused by _____-dependent activation of airway mast cells.

22. List four symptoms that, in an acute state, the asthmatic patient will exhibit.

    a. _____

    b. _____

    c. _____

    d. _____

AEROSOLIZED CORTICOSTEROIDS

23. What are the two most common methods used for the delivery of inhaled corticosteroids?

    a. _____

    b. _____

24. What is the approximant measured lung deposition of QVAR RediHaler?

25. How do fluticasone furoate and fluticasone propionate differ? How does this difference effect dosing?

26. What indicates good lung absorption of flunisolide?

27. List two available forms of Flovent.

    a. _____

    b. _____

28. What is the benefit of using budesonide in the form of Pulmicort Respules compared with the DPI Pulmicort?

29. What infection is reduced in patients that take ciclesonide?

30. What two drugs are contained within the dry powder inhaler (DPI) Advair?

    a. _____

    b. _____

31. What two drugs make up Symbicort?

    a. _____

    b. _____

32. What are oral inhalation and intranasal administration of glucocorticoids typically used to treat?

PHARMACOLOGY OF CORTICOSTEROIDS

33. Steroids suppress the inflammatory response by what three general pathways?

    a. _____

    b. _____

    c. _____

34. Besides suppression of the inflammatory response, what is another benefit of steroids?

HAZARDS AND SIDE EFFECTS OF STEROIDS

35. List six side effects associated with systemic administration of corticosteroids.

    a. _____

    b. _____

    c. _____

    d. _____

    e. _____

    f. _____

36. List three ways to minimize the local side effects of inhaled steroid administration.

    a. _____

    b. _____

    c. _____

CLINICAL APPLICATION

Use of Corticosteroids in Chronic Obstructive Pulmonary Disease

37. What are the different patterns in the inflammatory cells in chronic obstructive pulmonary disease (COPD) and those in asthma?

38. In asthma, to verify peak expiratory flow rate what devise should be used?

39. To enhance lung deposition what should a patient use when a patient is using a metered dose inhaler (MDI) for inhaled corticosteroids?

40. List five respiratory care assessments you would perform before the treatment of an inhaled corticosteroid.

    a. _____

    b. _____

    c. _____

    d. _____

    e. _____

41. List two respiratory care assessments you would perform with long-term treatment of an inhaled corticosteroid.

    a. _____

    b. _____

42. What three medications are contained in Trelegy Ellipta?

NATIONAL BOARD OF RESPIRATORY CARE (NBRC) TESTING QUESTIONS

1. Corticosteroids are naturally secreted by which of the following?
   a. Thymal cortex: outer zone
   b. Adrenal cortex: outer zone
   c. Adrenal cortex: inner zone
   d. Thymal cortex: inner zone

2. Which of the following are clinical indicators for intranasal aerosol steroids?
   1. Seasonal allergies
   2. Acute persistent mild asthma
   3. Perennial allergies
   4. Acute exacerbation of COPD
      a. 1 and 3 only
      b. 2 and 4 only
      c. 1, 2, and 3 only
      d. 2, 3, and 4 only

3. Corticosteroids are described as which of the following?
   a. Bronchodilators
   b. Smooth muscle dilators
   c. Anti-inflammatory agents
   d. Lipid-soluble agents

4. Which of the following occurs during an asthma attack?
   1. Bronchospasm
   2. Release of epinephrine
   3. Mucosal edema
   4. Increased secretions
      a. 1 and 4 only
      b. 2 and 3 only
      c. 1, 3, and 4 only
      d. 2, 3, and 4 only

5. Fluticasone propionate and salmeterol are drugs that are found in:
   a. Azmacort
   b. Advair HFA
   c. Symbicort
   d. QVAR

6. Which of the following are general symptoms of inflammation?
   1. Redness
   2. Swelling
   3. Heat
   4. Pain
      a. 1 and 2 only
      b. 3 and 4 only
      c. 2, 3, and 4 only
      d. 1, 2, 3, and 4

7. Regardless of the type of asthma, allergic or nonallergic, the major effector cells of the inflammatory response are which of the following?
   1. Neutrophil
   2. Mast cell
   3. Macrophage
   4. Eosinophil
      a. 1 and 3 only
      b. 2 and 4 only
      c. 1, 3, and 4 only
      d. 1, 2, and 4 only

8. Which of the following describes aerosol administration of corticosteroids?
   a. It is associated with no side effects.
   b. It produces severe side effects.
   c. It results in more systemic than local side effects.
   d. It results in minimal side effects

9. Which of the following is likely to increase local side effects associated with use of inhaled corticosteroids?
   a. Use of a spacer device
   b. Rinsing the mouth after each treatment
   c. Taking the lowest dose possible
   d. Taking the highest dose possible

10. Which of the following is recommended to avoid complicating side effects seen with systemic treatment with steroids?
    a. Reduce dosage
    b. Reduce number of days of treatment
    c. Switch to aerosol administration
    d. Switch to every-other-day administration

11. Early asthmatic response is caused by:
    a. Eosinophils
    b. Neutrophils
    c. Plasma leakage
    d. Immunoglobulin E

12. The common side effects of inhaled steroids include:
    1. Oral thrush
    2. Excessive oral secretions
    3. Dysphonia
    4. Yellowing of the teeth
       a. 2 and 4 only
       b. 1 and 3 only
       c. 1, 2, and 3 only
       d. 2, 3, and 4 only

13. Symbicort is a combination of:
    a. Albuterol and fluticasone
    b. Budesonide and formoterol
    c. Atrovent and fluticasone
    d. Budesonide and salmeterol

14. If a drug such as flunisolide shows a peak plasma level quickly, within 2 minutes, this would indicate:
    a. Reduced removal from the body by the kidney
    b. Excessive dose delivery
    c. Excessive oropharyngeal deposition
    d. Good absorption by the lungs

15. Mometasone and formoterol are drugs found in:
    a. Dulera
    b. Symbicort
    c. Advair
    d. QVAR

16. One of the primary reasons for using aerosolized glucocorticoids is to minimize _____ suppression.
    a. Eosinophil
    b. Neutrophil
    c. Adrenal
    d. White blood cell

17. A patient who has severe asthma has been prescribed corticosteroids for her treatment. She wants to know which type of corticosteroid she should use that will have minimal adverse effects. You would suggest:
    1. Inhaled
    2. Systemic
    3. Pill
    4. Injection
        a. 1 only
        b. 1 and 2 only
        c. 1, 3, and 4 only
        d. 1, 2, and 4 only

18. What is one advantage of using ciclesonide over other inhalation steroids?
    a. It decreases the development of *Candida albicans* in the mouth.
    b. It has a greater percent deposition in the lung.
    c. It is flavored and therefore reduces irritability in the oral cavity.
    d. It comes with a built-in holding chamber.

19. The best way to monitor changes in peak expiratory flow rate in a person with asthma who is taking inhaled steroids is to:
    a. Measure monthly steroid levels
    b. Keep a journal detailing nocturnal sleeping pattern
    c. Use a peak flow meter
    d. Use 1 month on and 1 month off treatment to identify wheezing patterns

20. To prevent the need to increase inhaled corticosteroid use in a person who is currently receiving low-dose inhaled steroids, which of the following is recommended?
    a. Short-term course of antibiotics
    b. Systemic corticosteroid administration
    c. Short-acting anticholinesterase medication
    d. Long-acting β_2 agonist

CASE STUDY 1
Asthma

Mrs. Peacock has been prescribed beclomethasone dipropionate (QVAR) 40 mcg/puff (two puffs two times daily) as treatment for moderate asthma.

1. How much QVAR will she receive in a 24-hour period?

2. Mrs. Peacock has never used an MDI with a spacer device. When you are instructing her in the use of her MDI, what points must you cover?

3. Mrs. Peacock wants to know whether she should increase the number of puffs of QVAR if she begins having shortness of breath and more coughing and wheezing. What do you tell her?

CASE STUDY 2
Asthma

(Information on the NAEPP can be accessed at http://www.nhlbi.nih.gov/guidelines/asthma/index .htm)

Zach is a 29-year-old male with asthma who lives in Atlanta. It is springtime, so the pollen is extremely thick. He monitors himself and is considered at present to require step 1 care in his management of asthma. When he has minor exacerbations, he uses his MDI of albuterol. Over the past 2 weeks, he has had several more exacerbations. His symptoms include nighttime coughing, increased wheezing, and tightness in his chest, and his peak expiratory flow rate has dropped 22%. He has come to the doctor's office, and the asthma educator sees him.

1. What should the educator recommend to Zach?

Zach has agreed to this change. It is now 4 days later and he is not getting better. In fact, his nighttime symptoms are worse, and he is not able to sleep through the night because of severe coughing. Seeking advice, he calls the asthma educator.

2. What is the next recommendation for Zach?

3. Zach has never taken the medication recommended in question 2. What would you tell him about the formulation and dosage?

CASE STUDY 3
Chronic Obstructive Lung Disease

(Information on the Global Initiative for Chronic Obstructive Lung Disease [GOLD] guidelines can be accessed at http://www.goldcopd.com/)

Charles is a 69-year-old patient in the emergency department who has complaints of increasing shortness of breath and increased coughing with increased sputum production. His sputum is more purulent in appearance, and he has a fever. His respiratory rate is 34 breaths/min, and his SpO_2 is 90%. He is taking albuterol by MDI at home. He states that he used his MDI but continues to be short of breath. His past medical history includes that he was a coal miner for 10 years and then became a laborer, cutting wood in a lumber yard. He has been admitted to the hospital several times over the past 5 years. He further states he used to smoke but gave that up a year ago. After the respiratory therapist and doctor have talked, they agree that the patient has COPD.

1. In this scenario, list four assessments that would indicate the patient may have COPD.

   a. _____

   b. _____

   c. _____

   d. _____

2. A laboratory report from a sample drawn earlier on admission has returned. Based on this patient's history, what would you expect would be a common inflammatory cell in this laboratory report?

3. Charles has been prescribed an inhaled corticosteroid after he is admitted to the hospital. He wants to know whether the corticosteroid will help his pulmonary function. What do you tell him?

4. Charles has been admitted to the hospital and has had a pulmonary function testing. Andy has been diagnosed with stage 2 moderate COPD. What are the three characteristics of stage 2 moderate COPD?

   a. _____

   b. _____

   c. _____

5. After several days, Charles is discharged. What respiratory home medications should he use to prevent future exacerbations?

6. Besides the respiratory home medications, what other pharmacologic treatment should be recommended based on his diagnosis and his age?

12 Nonsteroidal Antiasthma Agents

CHAPTER OUTLINE

Key Terms and Definitions
Identification of Nonsteroidal Antiasthma Agents
National Board of Respiratory Care (NBRC) Testing Questions
Case Study

CHAPTER OBJECTIVES

After answering the following questions, the reader should be able to:

1. Discuss the indications for nonsteroidal antiasthma agents
2. List available nonsteroidal antiasthma agents used in respiratory therapy
3. Differentiate between the specific nonsteroidal antiasthma agents
4. Describe routes of administration available for various nonsteroidal antiasthma agents
5. Describe the mechanism of action for various nonsteroidal antiasthma agents
6. Discuss the use of nonsteroidal antiasthma agents in the treatment of asthma

KEY TERMS AND DEFINITIONS

Complete the following questions by writing the answer in the space provided.

1. What is the term used to describe connective tissue cells that contain heparin and histamine?

2. What type of medication is Cromolyn?

3. What is the term used to describe chemical mediators that cause inflammation?

4. What is the term used to describe an agent that blocks the inflammatory response in asthma?

IDENTIFICATION OF NONSTEROIDAL ANTIASTHMA AGENTS

5. Which gamma globulin is produced by cells in the respiratory tract?

6. Alternatives to low-dose corticosteroids in step 2 asthma include what two types of medications?

7. What medication can be used for infants and children as an alternative to inhaled corticosteroids in step 2 asthma because of their safety profiles?

8. What term is used to describe nonsteroidal antiasthma that are not used during an acute exacerbation of asthma?

9. Describe a clinical situation in which the use of a controller medication is indicated.

10. The following is a list of drugs that are either controllers or relievers. *Place a C next to the drug if it is a controller and an R if it is a reliever.*

   a. Inhaled corticosteroids: _____

   b. Oral corticosteroids: _____

   c. Leukotriene modifiers: _____

   d. Cromolyn sodium: _____

   e. Inhaled short-acting β_2 agonists: _____

11. List three components of asthma.

   a. _____

   b. _____

   c. _____

12. List three modes of action of cromolyn sodium.

   a. _____

   b. _____

   c. _____

13. How many weeks of cromolyn sodium use is typically needed before reducing the concomitant therapy of bronchodilator or steroid use?

14. Does cromolyn sodium have any bronchodilating action?

15. Besides its use in asthma, list two other indications for the use of cromolyn.

   a. _____

   b. _____

16. Name two antileukotriene agents that have been approved for use in the United States.

   a. _____

   b. _____

17. What is the indication for Zileuton (Zyflo)?

18. What age is Zyflo is approved for use?

19. What is the recommended dosage of Zyflo for asthma?

20. What two important drugs in respiratory care does Zyflo interacts with?

Chapter **12** **Nonsteroidal Antiasthma Agents**

21. Accolate is indicated for prophylaxis and long-term treatment of asthma and has been approved for use in children of what age?

22. What is the mechanism of action for Accolate?

23. What is the dose of Accolate for children 5 to 11 years of age? 12 and older?

24. How should you instruct the child to take Accolate?

25. What is the minimum age Singulair is approved for?

26. How is Singulair available?

27. How is Singulair metabolized and excreted?

28. In moderate asthma, a combination of which medications results in greater lung function?

29. List the triggers for which antileukotrienes are particularly useful in controlling asthma.

    a. _____

    b. _____

    c. _____

30. Asthma guidelines agree that _____ are the most effective anti-inflammatory drugs for use in asthma, and they have broader anti-inflammatory activity than the more limited effect of the antileukotrienes.

31. A link appears to exist between respiratory syncytial virus (RSV) and asthma. The use of _____ blocks these mediators in asthma, as well as in RSV infection.

32. Briefly describe the mechanism of action of omalizumab (Xolair).

33. True or False: Xolair is not a replacement for corticosteroids.

34. True or False: Xolair is a prophylactic agent for uncontrolled moderate to severe persistent asthma.

35. True or False: Asthma rescue agents may need to be increased with the use of Xolair.

36. List seven advantages of antileukotriene drug therapy.

    a. _____

    b. _____

    c. _____

    d. _____

    e. _____

    f. _____

    g. _____

37. List six disadvantages of antileukotriene drug therapy.

   a. _____

   b. _____

   c. _____

   d. _____

   e. _____

   f. _____

38. List five monoclonal antibodies (Genaric name, Trade name)

   a. _____

   b. _____

   c. _____

   d. _____

   e. _____

NATIONAL BOARD OF RESPIRATORY CARE (NBRC) TESTING QUESTIONS

1. If a patient experiences an asthma attack as a result of exposure to cats, the asthma would be categorized as which of the following?
   a. Intrinsic
   b. Extrinsic
   c. Autoimmune
   d. Intangible

2. Airway obstruction that occurs with asthma is the result of:
   1. Bronchoconstriction
   2. Mucosal swelling
   3. Increased secretion production
   4. Excessive blood flow to the lungs
      a. 1 and 2 only
      b. 2 and 4 only
      c. 1, 2, and 3 only
      d. 2, 3, and 4 only

3. Release of cytokines during an allergic response does which of the following?
   a. Cytokines release B lymphocytes.
   b. Cytokines cause sloughing and death of eosinophils.
   c. Endothelial adhesion molecules are upregulated.
   d. Pulmonary vascular resistance is increased and leads to vascular congestion.

Chapter **12** Nonsteroidal Antiasthma Agents

4. Which of the following is a mast cell stabilizer?
   1. Cromolyn sodium
   2. Montelukast
   3. Zatirlukast
   4. Omalizumab
      a. 1 only
      b. 2 and 4 only
      c. 1, 2, and 3 only
      d. 2, 3, and 4 only

5. Cromolyn sodium is used to prevent which of the following?
   a. Inflammatory response
   b. Excessive accumulation of eosinophils
   c. Intrinsic asthma
   d. Reduction of nitric oxide response to asthma

6. The mechanism of action for Accolate is considered to be which of the following?
   a. 5-Lipoxygenase (5-LO) inhibitor
   b. Mast cell stabilizer
   c. Leukotriene receptor antagonist
   d. Leukotriene receptor agonist

7. Cromolyn can be used for the treatment of which of the following?
   a. Exacerbation of chronic obstructive pulmonary disease (COPD)
   b. Seasonal rhinitis
   c. Angiotensin-converting enzyme inhibitor (ACEI)-induced cough
   d. Flu-like symptoms within 2 days of onset

8. The ampoule or vial of cromolyn sodium contains 20 mg or 2 mL of aqueous solution, which is what percent solution?
   a. 1
   b. 2
   c. 3
   d. 4

9. You have determined extubation is not possible, owing to glottis swelling. The physician asks for your suggestion regarding medication choices, which will be given now to aid in the extubation process, which will happen tomorrow. What would you suggest?
   a. Metered dose inhaler (MDI) corticosteroids via endotracheal tube (ETT)
   b. Corticosteroids via oral gastric tube
   c. Intravenous corticosteroids
   d. MDI albuterol

10. Omalizumab (Xolair) can be given to children:
    a. 0 to 4 years of age
    b. 5 to 11 years of age
    c. 12 years of age or older
    d. Any age with approval from treating physician

11. For cromolyn sodium, it may take _____ to _____ weeks for improvement in patients' symptoms, allowing a decrease in concomitant therapy, such as bronchodilator or steroid use.
    a. 1 to 3
    b. 2 to 4
    c. 4 to 6
    d. 8 to 9

12. The antileukotriene modifier that is approved for children younger than 5 years of age is:
    a. Zyflo
    b. Singulair
    c. Accolate
    d. Xolair

13. Which of the following should be monitored once per month when taking Zyflo?
    a. Nitric oxide
    b. Liver enzymes
    c. Kidney enzymes
    d. Pulmonary function tests

14. Drugs that interact with Zyflo and may require dosing adjustment of Zyflo include:
    1. Theophylline
    2. Beclomethasone
    3. Cromolyn sodium
    4. Warfarin
        a. 1 and 4 only
        b. 2 and 3 only
        c. 1 and 2 only
        d. 2 and 4 only

15. For treatment of chronic asthma, a combination of _____ and _____ results in greater lung function than when these drugs are taken separately.
    a. β_2 Agonist and steroid
    b. β_2 Agonist and cromolyn sodium
    c. Corticosteroid and antileukotriene
    d. β_2 Agonist and antileukotriene

16. Concerning exercise-induced asthma, which of the following promotes the generation of leukotrienes that result in bronchoconstriction?
    a. Cooling and drying of the airway
    b. Increased blood flow to the lungs
    c. Airflow increase irritating goblet cells
    d. Increased body temperature producing excessive mucus production

17. Antileukotrienes are particularly useful in controlling asthma resulting from certain triggers, including which of the following?
    1. Exercise-induced asthma
    2. Aspirin-induced asthma
    3. Allergen-induced asthma
    4. Intrinsic-specific trigger asthma
        a. 1 and 2 only
        b. 2 and 4 only
        c. 1, 2, and 3 only
        d. 2, 3, and 4 only

18. Which of the following foods does the manufacturer recommend that montelukast granules be mixed with when given to a child?
    1. Breast milk
    2. Applesauce
    3. Carrots
    4. Rice
        a. 1 and 2 only
        b. 2 and 4 only
        c. 1, 2, and 3 only
        d. 1, 2, 3, and 4

19. Cromolyn prevents the extrusion of granules containing mediators of inflammation to the cell exterior. For this reason, cromolyn is referred to as a:
    1. Goblet cell inhibitor
    2. Nitric oxide stabilizer
    3. Protease inhibitor
    4. Mast cell stabilizer

20. Which of the following is a potent vasodilator that can damage cells and contribute to epithelial damage in asthma?
    a. Neurobinin A
    b. Nitric oxide
    c. Neurobinin B
    d. Neuropeptide

CASE STUDY

Todd is a 3-year-old boy who is in the doctor's office today for evaluation of his asthma. His asthma has been diagnosed as mild to moderate, and he uses a β agonist. After his evaluation, the doctor has decided to put Todd on a medication to help control his asthma. After discussing this with his mother, the doctor sends them to the asthma educator in the office for further consultation.

1. You are the asthma educator; what medication would you recommend for Todd? Why?

2. Because Todd is also receiving a bronchodilator by small-volume nebulizer, his mom asks whether a small-volume nebulizer can also give the medication, because it would be easiest, given that Todd has difficulty swallowing tablets. What would you tell her?

3. What instruction would you give his mother about how Todd could take this medication?

4. Todd's mom also would like to know whether there is a specific time of the day that Todd should take this medication. What would you tell her?

13 Aerosolized Anti-Infective Agents

CHAPTER OUTLINE

Key Terms and Definitions
Clinical Indications for Aerosolized Anti-Infective Agents
National Board of Respiratory Care (NBRC) Testing Questions
Case Studies 1 and 2

CHAPTER OBJECTIVES

After answering the following questions, the reader should be able to:

1. Define terms that pertain to aerosolized anti-infective agents
2. Discuss the indications for inhaled anti-infective agents
3. List all available inhaled anti-infective agents used in respiratory therapy
4. Differentiate between the specific anti-infective agent formulations
5. Discuss the route of administration available for the various anti-infective agents
6. Describe the mechanism of action for the various anti-infective agents
7. Recognize side effects for the various anti-infective agents
8. Discuss the use of each anti-infective agent in the treatment of lung disease

KEY TERMS AND DEFINITIONS

Complete the following questions by writing the answer in the space provided.

1. What does the term virostatic mean?

2. What virus causes formation of syncytial masses in infected cell structures?

3. Define Cystic Fibrosis.

4. What is a pneumonia common among patients with a lowered immune system response? What is the organism that causes it?

5. What does the term virucidal mean?

6. Define virus.

7. What is the indication for the following anti-infective agents? Also give the brand name.

   a. Pentamidine: _____, _____

   b. Ribavirin: _____, _____

   c. Tobramycin: _____, _____, _____

   d. Zanamivir: _____, _____

   e. Aztreonam: _____, _____

   f. Palivizumab: _____, _____

8. What type of agent is pentamidine?

9. In patients with acquired immunodeficiency syndrome (AIDS), what is the normal treatment dose and route of pentamidine?

10. What is the name of the nebulizer system recommended for use with pentamidine administration?

11. What is the flow rate used with the Respirgard II nebulizer system?

12. What mass median diameter (MMD) range of particles should be used for the effective nebulization of pentamidine?

13. What is the most common local side effect from aerosol administration of pentamidine?

14. When is aerosolized ribavirin indicated for use in the clinical setting?

15. What is the dose of ribavirin administered by the small-particle aerosol generator (SPAG)-2 nebulizer system?

16. When using a SPAG-2 nebulizer system in line with a mechanical ventilator, what should the respiratory therapist consistently monitor?

17. What is the reason for nearly continuous nebulization of ribavirin?

18. Give one example of a side effect of ribavirin that is associated with the following:

    a. Pulmonary: _____

    b. Cardiovascular: _____

    c. Dermatologic/topical: _____

19. What is the indication for Palivizumab (Synagis)?

20. What is the route of administration and frequency of Palivizumab?

21. Why is aerosolized tobramycin (TOBI) used with patients diagnosed with cystic fibrosis (CF)?

    a. _____

    b. _____

22. How can TOBI be administered to patients?

    a. _____

    b. _____

23. True or False: TOBI should be taken before other therapies, including chest physical therapy and bronchodilator therapy, to achieve the greatest airway clearance of secretions.

24. True or False: TOBI can be mixed with dornase alfa to achieve a synergistic effect.

25. Is a specific nebulizer and compressor system recommended for delivery of TOBI? If yes, what is it?

26. What is the dose and frequency for delivery of aerosolized TOBI?

27. What is the clinical use of inhaled aztreonam (Cayston)?

28. What medication should the patient be pretreated with before delivery of Cayston?

29. True of False. Cayston may also be used for patients with CF who are infected with *Burkholderia cepacia.*

30. _____ is an antiviral agent approved for use in the treatment of influenza in adults and children more than 5 years of age within the first 2 days of infection.

31. Before treating a patient with an aerosolized anti-infective, what must you do?

32. True or False: A short-acting β agonist can be given to prevent bronchospasm associated with administration of pentamidine.

33. True or False: When administering ribavirin to a child receiving mechanical ventilation, the respiratory therapist should consistently monitor in-line filters for obstruction resulting from drug precipitate.

34. True or False: Before administering aerosolized TOBI, the patient should be instructed that other inhaled medications should be taken.

35. True or False: A patient using zanamivir dry powder inhaler (DPI) should not use a bronchodilator if airway irritation causes bronchospasm.

120

1. Pentamidine is considered to be which of the following?
   a. Antifungal
   b. Antiparasitic
   c. Antiprotozoal
   d. Antibacterial

2. Pentamidine may be administered by which of the following routes of administration?
   1. Oral
   2. Inhalation
   3. IV
   4. Suppository
      a. 1 and 4 only
      b. 2 and 3 only
      c. 1, 2, and 3 only
      d. 2, 3, and 4 only

3. The only device currently approved by the U.S. Food and Drug Administration for the administration of pentamidine (NebuPent) is which of the following?
   a. SPAG-2
   b. Respirgard II
   c. AeroTech II
   d. Pari LC Plus

4. Small-volume nebulizers (SVNs) used to deliver pentamidine should be equipped with which of the following?
   1. Inspiratory filter
   2. Expiratory filter
   3. One-way valves
   4. Compression generators
      a. 3 and 4 only
      b. 2 and 3 only
      c. 1 and 2 only
      d. 1, 2, and 4 only

5. Ribavirin is classified as which of the following?
   a. Antiprotozoal
   b. Antifungal
   c. Antibacterial
   d. Antiviral

6. Which of the following is the clinical indication for ribavirin?
   a. Prophylactic treatment of *Pneumocystis jiroveci* pneumonia (PJP)
   b. Treatment of respiratory synctial virus (RSV) infection
   c. Treatment of chronic *Pseudomonas aeruginosa* infection
   d. Treatment of noninfluenza virus infection

7. For effective nebulization of pentamidine, the MMD of particles should be in the range of:
   a. 1 to 2 μm
   b. 3 to 4 μm
   c. 5 to 8 μm
   d. 1 to 10 μm

8. The standard dose of ribavirin administered by the SPAG-2 nebulizer system is:
   a. 10 mg/mL
   b. 20 mg/mL
   c. 30 mg/mL
   d. 35 mg/mL

Chapter **13 Aerosolized Anti-Infective Agents**

9. How should tobramycin be nebulized?
   a. Mixed with a short-acting beta agonist
   b. At the beginning of the aerosolized medication treatment regimen
   c. As a single agent in an approved nebulizer
   d. As a liquid nebulized solution in the TOBI Podhaler

10. Which of the following are indications for Cayston use in patients with CF?
    1. To treat influenza type B infections
    2. To treat and prevent early colonization of *P. aeruginosa*
    3. To maintain present lung function
    4. To reduce the rate of deterioration of lung function
       a. 1 and 2 only
       b. 1 and 3 only
       c. 2, 3, and 4 only
       d. 1, 2, and 4 only

11. Which of the following nebulizers is recommended for use to administer TOBI?
    a. SPAG-2
    b. Respirgard II
    c. Aerojet III
    d. PARI LC Plus

12. In what other disease can TOBI be used to treat *P. aeruginosa* infections?
    a. RSV
    b. Bronchiolitis
    c. Congenital heart disease
    d. No other diseases at this time

13. Which of the following statements is *true* regarding TOBI?
    a. Chest physical therapy should be administered as the patient is breathing TOBI.
    b. Dornase alfa may be mixed with TOBI to achieve a synergistic effect.
    c. TOBI should be administered after administration of all other therapy or medications.
    d. TOBI should be mixed with a short-acting β agonist to prevent bronchospasm.

14. A treatment dose of _____ mg of zanamivir is recommended for influenza infection.
    a. 5
    b. 10
    c. 20
    d. 200

15. Which of the following is the reason that ribavirin is administered for 12 to 18 hours per day for the treatment of RSV?
    a. A large quantity of drug rainout occurs because of the large particles formed from the SPAG-2 device.
    b. The powder creates increased rainout of the drug within the SPAG-2 nebulizer system.
    c. The drug has a short half-life in respiratory secretions.
    d. The liver metabolizes the drug quickly.

16. During the short-term respiratory care of a patient receiving TOBI, what assessments should occur?
    1. Monitor lung function
    2. Assess for improvement in weight
    3. Evaluate changes in hearing
    4. Monitor for signs of RSV
       a. 1 and 3 only
       b. 2 and 4 only
       c. 1, 2, and 3 only
       d. 2, 3, and 4 only

17. What is a clinical indication for the use of aztreonam (Cayston)?
    a. Forced expiratory volume at 1 second (FEV1) lower than 20%
    b. Pseudomonas aeruginosa colonization
    c. Staphylococcus aureus colonization
    d. Burkholderia cepacia colonization

18. Zanamivir (Relenza) is approved for children:
    a. Less than 1 year of age
    b. 2 to 3 years of age
    c. Greater than 5 years of age
    d. Greater than 12 years of age

19. Which of the following statements is *true* regarding administration of ribavirin in children?
    a. It should be administered immediately on diagnosis of routine RSV infection.
    b. It should be administered after 3 days of bronchodilator treatments have not been effective.
    c. It may be considered for life-threatening RSV infection.
    d. It should be considered only for children less than 6 months of age.

20. Oseltamivir phosphate (Tamiflu) has an off-label use for:
    a. Mild RSV
    b. H1N1 (swine flu)
    c. Bronchiolitis in infants with a history of prematurity
    d. RSV in infants with a history of congenital heart disease

CASE STUDY 1

Your patient, who was diagnosed with human immunodeficiency virus (HIV) in 1994, presents with a CD4$^+$ cell count of 100/mm^3, fever, shaking, chills, and productive cough. He has had PJP once before this admission and is allergic to trimethoprim-sulfamethoxazole (TMP-SMX). His diagnosis is PJP, and his physician has ordered pentamidine (NebuPent) treatments four times daily for treatment. As you do your pretreatment assessment, the patient tells you that he has previously been given pentamidine and that "It makes me cough pretty much throughout the whole treatment."

1. What do you recommend?

As a favor to you, one of your colleagues begins this treatment, using an SVN.

2. Should your colleague be using an SVN to administer pentamidine?

3. Other than using the Respirgard II, what precautions should you take to minimize your exposure to the pentamidine?

    a. _____

    b. _____

    c. _____

4. What adverse effects are you likeliest to suffer as a result of exposure to pentamidine?

Jeremy is a 7-year-old boy who has been in the hospital for the past 3 days for treatment of CF. He is being discharged, and his physician has ordered TOBI to be added to his pulmonary hygiene routine. Because this is the first time Jeremy will be taking TOBI, his parents have some questions. The physician has asked the respiratory therapist to meet with Jeremy and his parents to discuss the use of TOBI and to answer any other questions.

1. One of the first questions Jeremy's parents ask is: "What is TOBI, and why is he getting this drug?"

2. The next question is: "How much drug is Jeremy going to receive, and how often will he need to take it?"

3. His parents then ask: "Can this medication be nebulized in the same equipment that he is using for his dornase alfa and albuterol?"

4. His mother states: "Currently Jeremy takes his aerosolized medications with his Vest treatment. Can he just add the TOBI to his other medications as he does his Vest treatment? This really helps him in the morning to save time when he is getting ready to go to school."

5. His dad asks: "Does TOBI have any side effects?"

6. Jeremy and his parents are concerned about the voice alteration: "Is there anything that can be done to minimize it or prevent this from occurring?"

14   Antimicrobial Agents

CHAPTER OUTLINE

CHAPTER OBJECTIVES

After answering the following questions, the reader should be able to:

1. Define terms that pertain to antimicrobial agents
2. Define *antibiotic*
3. Describe the process involved in bacterial susceptibility testing
4. Discuss possible outcomes of antimicrobial combinations
5. List the various classes of penicillins
6. List the various classes of cephalosporins
7. Recognize similarities between members of macrolides, azalides, and ketolides
8. Recognize similarities between members of fluoroquinolones
9. List four mechanisms of action of antibacterials
10. List five commonly used antimycobacterials
11. Describe the commonly used azole antifungals and how they differ in spectrum of activity
12. Discuss similarities between members of echinocandins
13. Describe mechanisms of action of antiretrovirals

KEY TERMS AND DEFINITIONS

Complete the following by writing the answer in the space provided.

1. Define antimicrobial.

2. What term is used to describe when the combined effect of two antimicrobials is greater than their added effects?

3. Define antibiotics.

4. What term is used to describe when the effect of a combination of two antimicrobials is lower than the effect expected from either agent alone.

5. List four factors that should be considered before choosing an antimicrobial agent.

    a. _____

    b. _____

    c. _____

    d. _____

Identification of the Pathogen

6. What steps would need to be taken to identify the pathogen causing infection in a patient?

7. As a respiratory therapist, what is likely the most common specimen you will collect for culture?

8. What is the simplest and most common preparation by which to identify bacteria?

9. What color do Gram-positive bacteria stain? What color do gram-negative bacteria stain?

10. What is responsible for the difference in staining in a Gram stain?

11. *Mycobacterium tuberculosis* requires the use of what kind of stain to penetrate its wax-like cell wall?

12. Match the following common pathogens with their associated respiratory infection(s) in the adult.

    1. _____ Sinusitis

    2. _____ Community-acquired pneumonia (CAP)

    3. _____ Hospital-acquired pneumonia

    4. _____ Acute bronchitis

    5. _____ Cystic fibrosis (CF)

    a. *Staphylococcus aureus*
    b. *Mycoplasma pneumoniae*
    c. *Staphylococcus pneumoniae*
    d. *Haemophilus influenzae*
    e. *Streptococcus pneumoniae*

Susceptibility Testing and Resistance

13. Explain the *zone of inhibition* as it relates to susceptibility testing.

Host Factors

14. Describe a clinical situation where a patient may fail to respond to antimicrobial therapy.

15. Describe a clinical situation that may require adjustment of an antimicrobial drug dosage schedule.

16. What is the difference between bactericidal and bacteriostatic drugs?

Pharmacodynamics and Antimicrobial Combinations
17. Describe the postantibiotic effect.

18. How should two or more classes of antimicrobials are combined act?

MONITORING RESPONSE TO THERAPY

19. Although certain laboratory parameters can be monitored to assess the efficacy of an antimicrobial regimen, how is response to therapy is best measured?

ANTIBIOTICS

20. How do penicillins and cephalosporins exert their pharmacologic activity?

21. What type of antibiotics are carbapenems? What organism types are the effective against?

22. True or False: The monobactam aztreonam is active only against gram-negative aerobic bacilli such as *Pseudomonas aeruginosa*.

23. List two examples of aminoglycosides that are used in the treatment of cystic fibrosis (CF).

    a. _____

    b. _____

24. List three aminoglycosides that are used in the treatment of ventilator-associated pneumonia (VAP).

    a. _____

    b. _____

    c. _____

25. What broad-spectrum antibiotics are used in both pulmonary and systemic infections and are effective for treatment of diseases such as Rocky Mountain spotted fever, Lyme disease, and others?

26. What do tetracyclines inhibit that results in a bacteriostatic effect?

27. Vancomycin is useful for the treatment of infections caused by what organism?

28. What is one explanation for the increase in number of tuberculosis (TB) cases seen in recent years?

29. Patients with suspected TB should remain in their hospital room until one of the following three criteria is met. List all three.

a. _____

b. _____

c. _____

30. Treatment of tuberculosis consists of multiple antibiotics for how long?

31. How is *M. tuberculosis* is spread?

ANTIVIRAL AGENTS

32. What to antiviral agents (excluding antiretrovirals) do?

33. What antiviral agent is used against COVID-19?

BIOLOGICS

34. What is the current clinical use for biologics such as raxibacumab and obiltoxaximab?

NATIONAL BOARD OF RESPIRATORY CARE (NBRC) TESTING QUESTIONS

1. The simplest and most common preparation by which to identify bacteria is the:
   a. Acid-fast stain
   b. Gram stain
   c. Ziehl-Neelsen smear
   d. Agar plate count

2. Gram-positive bacteria stain _____, using the Gram stain method.
   a. Purple
   b. Red
   c. Pink
   d. Orange

3. An acid-fast stain is used to identify:
   a. *P. aeruginosa*
   b. *S. pneumoniae*
   c. *Candida* species
   d. *M. tuberculosis*

4. Which of the following common pathogens causes CAP?
   a. *S. aureus*
   b. *Mycobacterium pneumoniae*
   c. *P. aeruginosa*
   d. *H. influenzae*

5. A bacteriostatic drug is one that:
   a. Kills bacteria
   b. Inhibits bacterial growth
   c. Terminates replication
   d. Interferes with DNA replication

6. Although certain laboratory parameters can be monitored to assess efficacy of an antimicrobial regimen, response to therapy is best measured by:
   a. The number of antibiotics the patient is currently taking
   b. The strength of antibiotics the patient is currently taking
   c. The number of days the patient has been taking antibiotics
   d. Clinical assessment

7. Penicillins and cephalosporins exert their pharmacologic activity by inhibiting:
   a. Cell wall synthesis
   b. DNA replication
   c. RNA replication
   d. Viral replication

8. Broad-spectrum antibiotics are effective against:
   1. Viral infections
   2. Fungal infections
   3. Gram-positive infections
   4. Gram-negative infections
      a. 1 and 2 only
      b. 3 and 4 only
      c. 1, 2, and 4 only
      d. 2, 3, and 4 only

9. Which of the following aminoglycosides are used to treat CF?
   1. Amikacin
   2. Cephalosporins
   3. Tobramycin
   4. Tetracycline
      a. 2 and 4 only
      b. 1 and 3 only
      c. 3 and 4 only
      d. 1, 2, and 3 only

10. Which of the following drugs is used in the treatment of VAP?
    a. Erythromycin
    b. Tetracycline
    c. Fluoroquinolones
    d. Gentamicin

11. The drug of choice for *Legionella* bacteria is:
    a. Tetracycline
    b. Erythromycin
    c. Penicillin
    d. Gentamicin

12. Methicillin-resistant *S. aureus* (MRSA) is best treated with which of the following?
    a. Vancomycin
    b. Clindamycin
    c. Erythromycin
    d. Gentamicin

13. A patient suspected of having TB should remain in an isolation room until which of the following criteria is met?
    a. The patient is determined not to have TB.
    b. The patient has been pharmacologically treated for 5 days.
    c. The patient has three sputum samples obtained over a 3-day period.
    d. The patient no longer needs protective barriers, such as masks.

129

14. Drug treatment for tuberculosis consists of multiple antibiotics for:
    a. 5 to 7 days
    b. 12 to 15 days
    c. 1 to 2 months
    d. 6 to 12 months

15. Nosocomial transmission can be prevented by placing patients with suspected or confirmed tuberculosis in:
    a. Contact isolation
    b. Reverse isolation
    c. Respiratory isolation
    d. MRSA contact isolation

16. Initial therapy for treatment of TB involves a combination of which of the following medications?
    1. Isoniazid
    2. Pyrazinamide
    3. Rifampin
    4. Ethambutol
        a. 1 and 3 only
        b. 2 and 4 only
        c. 1, 2, and 4 only
        d. 1, 2, 3, and 4

17. Which of the following pathogens are commonly responsible for CAP?
    1. *S. pneumoniae*
    2. *H. influenzae*
    3. *M. pneumoniae*
    4. *Candidiasis albicans*
        a. 1 and 2 only
        b. 3 and 4 only
        c. 1, 3, and 4 only
        d. 1, 2, and 3 only

18. A sputum culture has returned and shows gram-negative bacilli (rods) present. This result would indicate:
    a. Colonization
    b. Hospital-acquired pneumonia
    c. Nosocomial pneumonia
    d. Aspiration pneumonia

19. Incidence of fungal infections has increased, and the most common species responsible for fungal infections is:
    a. *Scedosporium*
    b. *Candida*
    c. *Aspergillus*
    d. *Fusarium*

20. Which of the following are viral infections that would be treated with antiviral medications?
    1. Tuberculosis
    2. Herpes zoster
    3. Varicella-zoster
    4. Cytomegalovirus
        a. 1 and 3 only
        b. 2 and 4 only
        c. 1, 3, and 4 only
        d. 2, 3, and 4 only

Mr. Green lives in a homeless shelter in downtown Atlanta; he moved there from New Orleans after Hurricane Katrina. He has developed symptoms including a productive cough with blood-tinged sputum, chills, and sweating. He went to a local hospital emergency department, where he was diagnosed with TB.

1. What treatment regimen should be recommended for him?

2. Mr. Green has been admitted to the hospital. To prevent nosocomial transmission of TB, what would you suggest to provide respiratory isolation of this patient?

3. How long will Mr. Green have to remain in respiratory isolation?

4. What other measures should be recommended to health care employees entering Mr. Green's room that will help prevent the spread of *M. tuberculosis* by aerosolization?

Mrs. Palermo has been admitted to the hospital and is diagnosed with pneumonia. Physical assessment reveals a temperature of 38.5° C, a nonproductive cough, bibasilar crackles, and expiratory wheezing in all lung fields. Laboratory test results show an elevated white blood count (WBC). The respiratory therapist has been contacted to give breathing treatments and obtain a sputum sample for culture.

1. Many patients do not produce sputum with pneumonia, so what are common pathogens that cause pneumonia that may be considered for antibiotic therapy before obtaining a culture?

2. In the meantime, while waiting for a sputum sample for culture, what can be done to begin treating Mrs. Palermo's pneumonia?

3. After several breathing treatments, the patient produces enough sputum for culture. Analysis shows the patient to have an *S. pneumoniae* infection. What antibiotic could be helpful for this pathogen?

After several days of treatments, the patient's symptoms improve and WBC normalizes. The patient is sent home with several medications, including a 10-day supply of antibiotics, and is instructed to take all the medication. She also has an appointment to see her primary care physician in 2 weeks. Five days after being discharged from the hospital, Mrs. Palermo calls her primary care physician and explains that her temperature has returned, she is coughing and producing sputum, and she is feeling similar to when she entered the hospital.

4. What would you recommend asking the patient to help determine why her symptoms have returned?

15 Cold and Cough Agents

CHAPTER OBJECTIVES

After answering the following questions, the reader should be able to:

1. Define key terms that pertain to cold and cough agents
2. Differentiate between the common cold and the flu
3. Differentiate between the specific types of cold and cough agents
4. Discuss the mode of action for each specific cold and cough agent

KEY TERMS AND DEFINITIONS

Complete the following by writing the answer in the space provided.

1. Define antihistamine.

2. Describe the flu.

3. Define stimulant expectorants.

4. The best _____, especially with colds, is plain water and juices; caffeinated beverages, such as tea or colas, and beer or other alcoholic mixtures should be avoided.

5. Describe the common cold.

6. What are mucolytic expectorants? Give an example.

7. What are drugs that suppress the cough reflex, and are useful in the presence of an irritating, persistent, nonproductive cough called?

8. Match the following signs and symptoms of the common cold and influenza.

   1. _____ Fever   a. Cold
   2. _____ No chills present   b. Influenza
   3. _____ Headache
   4. _____ Nonproductive cough
   5. _____ Nasal congestion (common)
   6. _____ Early and severe fatigue
   7. _____ Sore throat (common)

9. Drugs that can cause rebound congestion if taken longer than a day and mimic the effects of the sympathetic nervous system are _____.

10. List four classes of drugs available to treat the common cold.

    a. _____

    b. _____

    c. _____

    d. _____

11. List the indications for each of the four classes listed in question 10.
    a. _____

    b. _____

    c. _____

    d. _____

SYMPATHOMIMETIC (ADRENERGIC) DECONGESTANTS

12. How long should adrenergic nasal sprays be used? Explain why.

13. Topical sympathomimetic _____ sprays or drops produce results faster than oral applications.

ANTIHISTAMINE AGENTS

14. Where are the following receptors located, and what does stimulation of each result in?

    a. H_1: _____

    b. H_2: _____

    c. H_3: _____

15. What are three effects of antihistamines?

    a. _____

    b. _____

    c. _____

16. The anticholinergic effect of first-generation H_1 receptor cold medications contributes to _____ _____ drying.

EXPECTORANTS

17. What are three ways stimulant expectorants work?

    a. _____

    b. _____

    c. _____

18. The best expectorant for a simple cold is _____.

19. How do bland aerosols of saline increase sputum volume?

    a. _____

    b. _____

COUGH SUPPRESSANTS (ANTITUSSIVES)

20. List a situation in which the use of antitussives would not be indicated.

21. A common narcotic cough suppressant is _____.

COLD COMPOUNDS: TREATING A COLD

Complete the following by writing the undesirable effects of each category of ingredient in the space provided.

22. Sympathomimetics

    a. _____

    b. _____

    c. _____

23. Antihistamines

    a. _____

    b. _____

    c. _____

24. Expectorants

    a. _____

25. Antitussives

    a. _____

NATIONAL BOARD OF RESPIRATORY CARE (NBRC) TESTING QUESTIONS

1. Which of the following agents is useful in the presence of an irritating, persistent, nonproductive cough?
   a. Antitussive
   b. Expectorant
   c. Mucolytic expectorant
   d. Sympathomimetic

2. An antihistamine used to treat a common cold is intended to:
   a. Decongest
   b. Suppress the cough reflex
   c. Dry secretions
   d. Increase mucus clearance

3. An agent that increases the production and clearance of mucus secretions in the respiratory tract is called a(n):
   a. Antihistamine
   b. Antitussive
   c. Mucolytic expectorant
   d. Stimulant expectorant

4. An alternative to antihistamines for rhinorrhea in a cold is the anticholinergic nasal spray:
   a. Spiriva
   b. Combivent
   c. Atrovent
   d. Albuterol

5. The common cold is usually _____ in origin.
   a. Bacterial
   b. Viral
   c. Fungal
   d. Allergenic

6. Which of the following is associated with "rebound congestion" concerning oral administration of sympathomimetic decongestants?
   a. Slower onset of action
   b. Better decongestion
   c. Increased systemic side effects
   d. Overuse of these agents

7. Which of the following classes of effects applies or apply to antihistamines?
   1. Antihistaminic
   2. Sedative
   3. Anticholinergic
   4. Sympathomimetic
      a. 4
      b. 2 and 3
      c. 1, 2, and 3
      d. 1, 3, and 4

8. The anticholinergic effect of antihistamines on the upper airway results in:
   a. Bronchoconstriction
   b. Capillary leakage
   c. Drying
   d. Increased mucus production

9. Which of the following is recommended as being safe and effective as an expectorant?
   a. Terpin hydrate
   b. Guaifenesin
   c. Glycerol
   d. Iodine

10. The best expectorant for a cold is:
    a. Water
    b. Terpin hydrate
    c. Guaifenesin
    d. Glycerol

11. Which of the following side effects is most associated with an antihistamine?
    a. Tremor
    b. Drowsiness
    c. Hypertension
    d. Tachycardia

12. Which of the following is best for a patient who has a nonproductive, irritating, dry, hacking cough?
    a. Expectorant
    b. Antihistamine
    c. Cough suppressant
    d. Sympathetic stimulant

13. Which of the following Robitussin medications would you want to avoid during the day while working or driving?
    a. Robitussin cold and cough
    b. Robitussin DAC
    c. Robitussin Cough and Allergy
    d. Robitussin Sneeze and Wheeze

14. A rational approach to surviving colds and preventing spread of rhinovirus is:
    1. Yearly flu shot
    2. Antibiotics
    3. Fluids
    4. Rest
       a. 1 and 2
       b. 2 and 4
       c. 3 and 4
       d. 2, 3, and 4

15. If a patient has cardiovascular problems and is using a decongestant, which of the following should be monitored for this patient?
    1. Blood pressure
    2. Oxygen saturation
    3. Temperature
    4. Heart rate
       a. 2 and 3
       b. 2 and 4
       c. 1, 2, and 4
       d. 2, 3, and 4

CASE STUDY 1

Your parents are away on a cruise and left you babysitting your little brother during spring break. Over the past few days, he has developed a runny nose, is sneezing, and says he feels "icky." You take his temperature and it is 98.8° F.

1. What is the most likely diagnosis?

2. What treatment would help him the most at present?

3. Being a good respiratory therapist, you anticipate that he may develop a cough that is dry and nonproductive, even though his temperature remains normal. You ask yourself: "Is there anything in his treatment regimen that can be changed so that I won't have to take him to the doctor?"

CASE STUDY 2

You are a respiratory therapist working for a home care company. You are visiting a patient, Mrs. Fields, to check on some equipment she is renting. While you are there, she tells you that she doesn't feel well. She says she felt fine 2 days ago, but today she has a nonproductive cough that keeps her awake at night, chills, headache, no energy, and aching muscles. She asks: "Do you think I have a cold?"

1. Based on her description of symptoms, what would you tell her?

2. What infectious agent may have caused this illness?

3. She says that the worst part about this illness is a dry, hacking, nonproductive cough that keeps her awake at night. She asks you whether there is something she can take that would stop her coughing so she can sleep. What would you tell her?

4. What precaution would you want to tell Mrs. Fields about taking this medication during the daytime?

16 Selected Agents of Pulmonary Value

CHAPTER OBJECTIVES

After answering the following questions, the reader should be able to:

1. Define key terms and definitions pertaining to selected agents of pulmonary value
2. Discuss the indication for α_1-proteinase inhibitor therapy
3. Recognize α_1-proteinase inhibitor deficiency in a patient
4. List available α_1-proteinase inhibitors
5. List three types of formulations for nicotine replacement therapy
6. Recognize the advantages and disadvantages of nicotine replacement and medications used for smoking cessation
7. Discuss the use of e-cigarettes as an adjunct or as an alternative to smoking cessation
8. Discuss the indication for nitric oxide
9. Describe the effect of inhaled nitric oxide on a patient
10. List the two toxic products of nitric oxide
11. List the two inhaled prostacyclin analogs available in the United States
12. Name the only inhaled insulin product available in the United States
13. Recognize the need for adding roflumilast to a patients continuum of care
14. Determine the need for adding Trikafta to a patient's treatment regime

KEY TERMS AND DEFINITIONS

Match the following definitions with their terms.

1. _____ α_1-Proteinase inhibitor (API) has altered electrophoretic properties and lower-than-normal serum concentrations.

2. _____ Also known as *α_1-proteinase inhibitor*, this inhibitor of trypsin may be deficient in patients with emphysema.

3. _____ Undetectable API levels in the serum.

4. _____ API is present in normal amounts but does not function normally.

5. _____ Individual has normal serum levels of API.

a. α_1-Antitrypsin (α_1-AT)
b. API deficient
c. API dysfunctional
d. API normal
e. API null

6. How is α_1-AT (Prolastin) prepared?

7. Describe how α_1-AT deficiency is similar to cystic fibrosis?

8. The enzyme neutrophil elastase, which can destroy alveolar walls, is held in check by _____.

9. Explain the pathogenesis of emphysema caused by α_1-AT deficiency.

10. What long-term replacement therapy is incidated for individuals with congenital deficiency of API?

11. True or False: Given the nature of the disease and the action of the drugs, α_1-AT proteinase-inhibiting drugs cannot reverse damage or improve lung function.

12. Indicate whether the following statements are either *True* or *False* concerning assessment of α_1-AT replacement therapy.
    a. True or False: Overall pulmonary health should be assessed, based on frequency and severity of respiratory infections, cough, sputum production if present, and hospitalization rate.
    b. True or False: Pulmonary function testing of flow rates is used to monitor the degree of airflow obstruction for short-term use of the drug.

13. What receptor does nicotine stimulates at the autonomic ganglia of both the sympathetic and parasympathetic nervous systems?

14. List seven physical symptoms a patient may experience during nicotine withdrawal.

    a. _____

    b. _____

    c. _____

    d. _____

    e. _____

    f. _____

    g. _____

15. List five forms of nicotine replacement.

    a. _____

    b. _____

    c. _____

    d. _____

    e. _____

16. What is the indication for nicotine replacement therapy? Who benefits most from therapy?

17. Explain why the nicotine inhaler may be preferred to gum and nasal spray.

18. _____ is an antidepressant found in Wellbutrin; it is also a nonnicotine aid to smoking cessation.

19. How does Chantix work?

20. What is a precaution you should explain to your patient that is receiving nicotine replacement therapy?

21. What antihypertensive agent has been prescribed to reduce symptoms of opioid and alcohol withdrawal?

22. How is Nitric oxide (NO) used in respiratory therapy?

23. What are the indications for inhaled nitric oxide (INO) in neonates?

24. What is the recommended dosage of INO?

25. Administration of INO at more than the recommended dose can cause increased levels of _____ _____ and _____.

26. According to the American Academy of Pediatrics, where should sample gas for analysis should be drawn?

27. True or False: Blood methemoglobin levels should be drawn every other day.

28. True or False: Weaning from NO should be gradual to prevent arterial desaturation and pulmonary hypertension.

29. True or False: The dose of NO should always start at 40 ppm and can be increased to 80 ppm if no clinical signs of pulmonary vasodilation occur.

30. True or False: Because INO has a short half-life, as soon as the INO is discontinued, pulmonary vasodilation ends.

31. What should institutions have the capacity to do in the event NO therapy fails?

32. List a contraindication to NO.

33. When does INO become inactive?

34. Some endogenous NO is exhaled from the lungs after being converted to _____ within the red blood cells.

35. Improvement of arterial oxygen pressure (Pao_2) with INO results from dilation of pulmonary blood vessels and improved _____ _____ matching.

36. NO is administered to an infant receiving _____ _____.

37. Preductal and postductal shunting can be monitoring during NO delivery by monitoring the _____.

38. Ventavis dilates _____ and _____ vascular beds when given via inhalation.

39. What two aerosol delivery systems are recommended for administration of Ventavis?

   a. _____

   b. _____

40. In patients with chronic obstructive pulmonary disease (COPD) receiving Ventavis, pretreatment with what medication may be beneficial to prevent bronchospasm?

41. Tyvaso is an inhaled prostacyclin vasodilator for the treatment of _____ _____.

42. Tyvaso should not be used in patients _____ years of age.

43. What is an indication for the use of Roflumilast?

44. During treatment and short term what respiratory care assessment should be performed on a patient taking a phosphodiesterase 4 inhibitor?

45. What precaution should be taken for patient taking a CFTR modulator?

1. What type of disorder is α_1-AT deficiency?
   a. Autosomal recessive
   b. Disomonal
   c. Trisomy 13
   d. XY recessive

2. Which statement is *true* regarding α_1-AT deficiency?
   a. It is generally seen at a later age, as a result of smoking.
   b. It is caused by excessive exposure to asbestos at an early age.
   c. It develops at an early age among people without cause (smoking, relevant work history).
   d. It develops predominantly in men more than 65 years of age with a history of exposure to wood dust.

3. Which of the following are signs of high physical addiction/dependence on nicotine?
   1. Smokes more than 5 cigarettes per day
   2. Smokes within 30 minutes of rising from bed
   3. Smokes even when bedridden from illness
   4. Smokes more frequently in the morning
      a. 1 and 4 only
      b. 1 and 3 only
      c. 1, 2, and 3 only
      d. 2, 3, and 4 only

4. What is the purpose of nicotine replacement therapy?
   a. To reduce the number of cigarettes smoked by a patient
   b. To reduce the food cravings of a smoking patient who is cutting down on the number of cigarettes smoked per day
   c. To replace the nicotine lost with smoking cessation
   d. To help eliminate nicotine from the body during weaning from cigarette smoking

5. Which of the following methods of administering nicotine would simulate a cigarette and give oral gratification?
   a. Nicotine gum
   b. Nicotine nasal spray
   c. Nicotine patch
   d. Nicotine inhaler

6. Bupropion contains which of the following?
   1. Nonnicotine agent to help reduce smoking
   2. Antidepressant
   3. Analgesic
   4. Nicotine
      a. 1 and 2 only
      b. 2 and 3 only
      c. 1 and 3 only
      d. 1, 2, and 3 only

7. Before prescribing varenicline (Chantix) to a patient who is currently smoking, you should have the patient set a quit date and start the medication _____ week(s) before this date.
   a. 1
   b. 2
   c. 3
   d. 4

8. The indication for INO is for neonates with a gestational age of:
   a. Greater than 34 weeks
   b. Greater than 24 weeks
   c. Less than 27 weeks
   d. Less than 31 weeks

9. INO is considered to be a selective pulmonary artery vasodilator because:
   a. It is inhaled
   b. The nitric oxide rapidly deactivates once it attaches to hemoglobin
   c. A large dose is administered and the oxygen concentration is high
   d. It converts to nitrogen dioxide, which remains in the lung

10. The recommended dose of INO is:
    a. 80 ppm
    b. 60 ppm
    c. 40 ppm
    d. 20 ppm

11. Administration of NO at more than the recommended levels can increase levels of:
    1. Methemoglobin
    2. Nitrogen dioxide
    3. Sulfhemoglobin
    4. Nitrohemoglobin
       a. 1 and 2 only
       b. 2 and 3 only
       c. 1, 3, and 4 only
       d. 2 and 4 only

12. Which of the following medications is used as a CFTR for patients with cystic fibrosis?
    a. Ventavis
    b. Tyvaso
    c. Roflumilast
    d. Ivacaftor

13. Use of bupropion is associated with a dose-dependent risk of:
    a. Bronchospasm
    b. Excessive secretions in lower airway
    c. Seizure
    d. Pulmonary artery vasoconstriction

14. Nicotine replacement therapy should be carefully weighed in patients with:
    a. Diabetes type 2
    b. Diabetes type 1
    c. Cardiovascular disease
    d. Asthma

15. According to the American Academy of Pediatrics, sampling of gas containing NO for analysis of a patient on mechanical ventilation should take place:
    a. On the inspiratory side of the patient circuit, where INO first enters the circuit
    b. On the expiratory side of the patient circuit
    c. Before the wye adaptor, proximal to the patient
    d. On the expiratory side of the patient circuit, just before the exhalation valve of the ventilator

16. Which of the following are indications for NO therapy for neonates?
    1. Hypoxic respiratory failure
    2. Lung hypoplasia
    3. Immature lungs and deficient surfactant
    4. Pulmonary hypertension
       a. 1 and 3 only
       b. 2 and 3 only
       c. 1 and 4 only
       d. 1, 3, and 4 only

17. NO is administered to an infant through which of the following?
    a. Nonrebreather mask
    b. High-flow nasal cannula
    c. Mechanical ventilation
    d. Bubble CPAP system

18. Preductal and postductal shunting can be monitored during NO delivery by monitoring which of the following?
    a. Capillary blood gases
    b. Umbilical venous blood gases
    c. Scalp venous blood gases
    d. Pulse oximetry measurement

19. Which of the following aerosol delivery systems is recommended for administration of iloprost (Ventavis)?
    a. Aerogen vibrating mesh
    b. Misty Neb
    c. Prodose ADD system
    d. MicroNeb

20. Prostinil (Tyvaso) is an inhaled prostacyclin vasodilator for the treatment of which of the following?
    a. Pulmonary hypertension
    b. Systemic hypotension
    c. Atrial fibrillation with associated systemic hypotension
    d. Premature ventricular contractions (more than six per minute) with pulmonary hypotension

CASE STUDY 1

You are conducting a smoking cessation class at a local pulmonary rehabilitation clinic. One of the participants is the president of a local university. Because she is new to the class, you interview her to obtain a smoking history and to see whether she has a high physical addiction to nicotine. Her history indicates the following:
    She works an average of 60 hours per week and is widely known throughout her community.
    She feels she has a high level of stress.
    She smokes a pack a day.
    She lights her first cigarette within 30 minutes of rising from bed in the morning.
    Her smoking occurs mostly in the morning, especially on her 1.5-hour commute to the university.
    Even though her campus is smoke-free, she admits to slipping out from her office to smoke.

1. Based on her interview, does she have a physical addiction to nicotine?

2. She asks you to recommend the smoking cessation method that would best suit her lifestyle. What would you recommend?

3. After some use of the transdermal patch, she complains that she has skin irritation where she places the patch each day. What would you recommend?

4. Your patient is a heavy smoker (approximately 20 cigarettes a day). What size patch (in milligrams) would be recommended for her level of smoking?

5. After 2 weeks on the transdermal patch, she complains of feeling depressed and feels she cannot continue with the smoking cessation program. What would you suggest?

CASE STUDY 2

A 35-week gestational age infant is currently intubated and receiving mechanical ventilation with an Fio_2 of 1.0 with a resulting Spo_2 of 80%. Echocardiography has been performed and indicates the presence of pulmonary hypertension. The decision has been made to begin therapy inline through the ventilator.

1. What is the recommended initial starting dose of NO?

2. The nurse is concerned about the newborn's systemic blood pressure during delivery of NO, because the baby's blood pressure is currently low. How would you respond to this concern?

3. After 20 minutes, the infant's Spo_2 has increased to 95%. What does this indicate that is occurring in the lungs?

4. A measurement of NO shows it to be 1%. Is this going to be a concern for the formation of methemoglobin?

The infant has now been on mechanical ventilation for 2 days. Currently, the infant is receiving 18 ppm, and the Fio_2 is 0.60 and Spo_2 is 94%. An order has been written to continue decreasing the NO in increments of 2 ppm. After the NO is decreased to 16 ppm, the Spo_2 drops to 83%.

Chapter **16** **Selected Agents of Pulmonary Value**

5. a. Why could this have occurred?

  b. What should be done to increase the Sp_{O_2}?

6. What formula could be used to evaluate the relationships among mean airway pressure of the ventilator, ventilator Fi_{O_2}, and Pa_{O_2}?

17 Neonatal and Pediatric Aerosolized Drug Therapy

CHAPTER OUTLINE

Key Terms and Definitions
Introduction
Off-Labeled Use of Drugs in Neonatal and Pediatric Patients
Factors Affecting Neonatal and Pediatric Aerosol Drug Delivery
Clinical Response to Aerosolized Drugs in Neonatal and Pediatric Patients
Selection of Delivery Devices
Compliance and Cooperation During Aerosol Therapy
Aerosol Administration in Intubated Neonatal and Pediatric Patients
National Board of Respiratory Care (NBRC) Testing Questions
Case Studies 1 and 2

CHAPTER OBJECTIVES

After answering the following questions, the reader should be able to:

1. Define key terms that pertain to neonatal and pediatric drug therapy
2. Explain off-label use of aerosolized medications in neonates and children
3. List and describe the most important factors affecting neonatal and pediatric aerosol drug delivery
4. Describe the clinical response of neonatal and pediatric patients to aerosolized drugs
5. Describe special circumstances related to selection of delivery devices for neonatal and pediatric patients
6. Explain the most relevant factors to select the appropriate aerosol delivery device according to age group
7. Describe the implications of compliance and cooperation on the efficiency of aerosol delivery
8. List some of the novel inhaled therapies under investigation for pediatric patients
9. Explain the importance of parent education in the administration of inhalation therapy to children
10. Explain lung deposition of inhaled drugs in pediatric and neonatal intubated patients

KEY TERMS AND DEFINITIONS

Match the following definitions with their terms.

1. _____ A child between the ages of 1 month and 1 year.

2. _____ The dose actually reaching the trachea and beyond.

3. _____ The period of time between birth and the first month of life.

4. _____ Refers to the period of time between 1 month and 18 years of age.

5. _____ The dose released by the aerosol device.

6. _____ The dose reaching the patient's mouth or artificial airway.

7. _____ The dose in the delivery device.

8. _____ Use of drugs with no U.S. Food and Drug Administration (FDA)–approved labeled use.

a. Emitted dose
b. Infant
c. Inhaled or delivered dose
d. Lung dose
e. Neonatal
f. Nominal dose
g. Off-label
h. Pediatric

9. In the neonatal and pediatric population, even when an optimal device is selected, what are three important factors that can reduce lung deposition?

   a. _____

   b. _____

   c. _____

10. In your own words, what is the "pediatric rule" as it relates to the FDA?

OFF-LABELED USE OF DRUGS IN NEONATAL AND PEDIATRIC PATIENTS

11. Is it legal for physicians to prescribe off-label use of drugs to pediatric patients?

12. Drug dosing with inhaled aerosols is not based on body size and blood level but on _____ _____.

13. *Fill in the following table,* indicating the differences between neonatal and adult anatomy and respiratory parameters that would affect aerosol penetration and deposition.

	Neonate	Adult
a. Tracheal length		
b. Tidal volume		
c. Minute ventilation		
d. Respiratory rate		
e. Inspiratory flow rate		

FACTORS AFFECTING NEONATAL AND PEDIATRIC AEROSOL DRUG DELIVERY

14. List three reasons that children inhale a smaller percentage of the emitted dose from either a small-volume nebulizer (SVN) or metered dose inhaler (MDI) with a reservoir device.

   a. _____

   b. _____

   c. _____

15. The following is a list of factors that may affect the dose inhaled from a reservoir chamber by neonatal and pediatric patients. *Identify each as either (1) a mechanical and design factor or (2) a patient factor.*

   a. _____ Electrostatic charge on plastic devices
   b. _____ Tidal volume
   c. _____ Presence of inspiratory valve
   d. _____ Inspiratory flow rate
   e. _____ Amount of dead volume in mouthpiece

   1. Mechanical and design factor

   2. Patient factor

16. A crying infant has _____ lung deposition and _____ gastrointestinal (GI) tract deposition.

17. Why may a younger patient (younger than 18 months of age) not have as great a clinical response to medication compared with an older child?

18. What outcome measures have documented clinical efficacy of aerosolized bronchodilators with infants?

SELECTION OF DELIVERY DEVICES

19. Name the current methods used to deliver therapeutic aerosols.

20. List the type of aerosol system that can be used for each of the age groups listed.

    a. Neonate: _____

    b. Child 5 years of age or older: _____

    c. Child 4 years of age or older: _____

    d. Child up to 4 years of age: _____

21. Although pressurized MDIs (pMDIs) may be routinely used, why may a nebulizer be a preferred method of delivery of aerosolized medication?

22. Why is a dry powder inhaler (DPI) not appropriate for children younger than 5 years?

COMPLIANCE AND COOPERATION DURING AEROSOL THERAPY

23. Applying a face mask to a child may cause crying. What are three effects produced by crying that will negatively affect aerosol delivery?

    a. _____

    b. _____

    c. _____

24. In one study, crying led to more extrathoracic aerosol deposition and greater risks of _____ _____.

25. Dose variability depends more on _____ and less on _____ design.

26. Explain why "blow-by" cannot be used with pMDIs.

27. How can smaller tidal volumes in pediatric patients be compensated when delivering medications via a pMDI with a valved holding chamber?

AEROSOL ADMINISTRATION IN INTUBATED NEONATAL AND PEDIATRIC PATIENTS

28. List three potential problems that may occur with an externally powered nebulizer placed inline on a pediatric and neonatal ventilator.

    a. _____

    b. _____

    c. _____

29. A _____/_____ nebulizer can be used inline with mechanical ventilation because it does not require external gas to power the nebulizer.

30. Most studies show a slightly higher lung deposition with the pMDI placed between the _____ piece and _____ _____.

31. Aerosol delivery may be less effective with _____ ventilation versus mechanical ventilation.

32. To improve lung deposition, the pMDI should be activated _____ _____.

NATIONAL BOARD OF RESPIRATORY CARE (NBRC) TESTING QUESTIONS

1. A person in the first 4 weeks of postnatal life is correctly termed which of the following?
   a. Postmature neonate
   b. Neonate
   c. Infant
   d. Baby

2. Why are SVNs not effective when treating infants with an inspiratory flow rate of less than 100 mL/sec?
   a. They would not completely inhale all of the nebulizer output during the inspiratory phase
   b. The noise is irritating to them
   c. They fall asleep before the treatment is over
   d. No research has been done to prove it works

3. Which aerosol delivery devices can be used to treat a 5-year-old patient?
   1. SVN
   2. MDI with spacer
   3. DPI
   4. Breath-actuated MDI
      a. 1 and 2
      b. 2 and 3
      c. 1, 3, and 4
      d. 1, 2, 3, and 4

4. Aerosol deposition in the neonate can be affected by which of the following?
   1. Increased inspiratory flow rate
   2. Smaller tidal volume
   3. Smaller airways
   4. Shorter respiratory cycle
      a. 1 and 2 only
      b. 2 and 3 only
      c. 1, 2, and 4 only
      d. 2, 3, and 4 only

5. Which of the following applies to a DPI?
   a. Requires that the user generates more than 60 L/min of flow
   b. Should be used only with a spacer
   c. Can be done with an endotracheal tube
   d. Can be used in the neonatal population

6. The dose of drug that is released from the aerosol device is called the:
   a. Inhaled dose
   b. Target dose
   c. Emitted dose
   d. Lung dose

7. Which of the following is the normal tidal volume for a neonate?
   a. 2 mL/kg
   b. 3 mL/kg
   c. 4 mL/kg
   d. 6 mL/kg

8. You are administering an SVN aerosol to a 9-year-old asthmatic child. The amount of albuterol you place in the SVN is called the:
   a. Nominal dose
   b. Lung dose
   c. Effective dose
   d. Target dose

9. The delivered dose of medication from an SVN, MDI, or DPI that actually reaches the trachea and beyond is the

   _____ dose.
   a. Emitted
   b. Lung
   c. Target
   d. Specific

10. The actual dose of an inhaled aerosol drug in neonates can be as low as:
    a. Less than 1%
    b. 5%
    c. 10%
    d. 15%

11. Which of the following patient factors affect the dose inhaled from a reservoir chamber?
    1. Inspiratory flow rate
    2. Tidal volume
    3. Respiratory cycle
    4. Position of the patient in bed
       a. 1 and 4 only
       b. 2 and 3 only
       c. 1, 2, and 3 only
       d. 2, 3, and 4 only

12. Administration of nebulized aerosol with a face mask using the "blow-by" technique can reduce the inhaled drug mass in a pediatric patient as much as:
    a. 50%
    b. 10%
    c. 5%
    d. 1%

13. Although pMDIs may be routinely used, a nebulizer is a preferred method of delivery of which of the following?
    a. Delivery of mucolytic agents
    b. Delivery of corticosteroids
    c. Delivery of leukotriene modifiers
    d. Delivery of hypertonic saline for cough induction

14. When using an externally powered nebulizer inline on a mechanical ventilator, which of the following are potential problems that can occur?
    1. Increased volume or pressure
    2. Bias flow interference with patient triggering
    3. Decreased levels of positive end-expiratory pressure (PEEP)
    4. Variable fraction of inspired oxygen (FiO_2)
       a. 1 only
       b. 2 and 3 only
       c. 1, 2, and 4 only
       d. 2, 3, and 4 only

15. To improve lung deposition of a patient receiving mechanical ventilation, when should the pMDI be activated?
    a. During inspiration
    b. At the end of expiration
    c. At the beginning of expiration
    d. Only during a spontaneous breath

CASE STUDY 1

A 4-month-old infant girl has been admitted to the hospital from the emergency department. The mother states her child has had a fever, persistent cough, and wheezing over the last 2 days. On assessment, the infant has a respiratory rate of 42 breaths/min, her pulse is 136 beats/min, and her temperature is 39° C. Further assessment reveals accessory muscle use and some nasal flaring. Auscultation findings include bilateral expiratory wheeze and coarse crackles in the upper lobes. The respiratory therapist suggests that the infant should receive aerosol therapy using albuterol.

1. What delivery devices are available to you?

2. Which method of delivery would you select? Justify your selection.

3. As you begin the treatment, she starts to cry and thrashes around on your lap, thus making it difficult for her to receive an effective treatment. What should you do?

4. Three days later, the child is doing much better and is being discharged. The child has been ordered to receive albuterol while at home. What delivery device should the respiratory therapist recommend for home use?

A 6-year-old child is in the intensive care unit and is receiving volume control mechanical ventilation.
The child has the following settings:

    Mode: Assist control
    Tidal volume: 150 mL
    Rate: 20/min
    PEEP: 5 cm H_2O
    Fio_2: 0.50

Respiratory assessment reveals bilateral expiratory wheezing with coarse crackles. Over the past
few hours, the pressure on the ventilator has steadily increased, indicating greater airway resistance.
The respiratory therapist, according to protocol, begins administering levalbuterol every 4 hours.

1. What formulation of FDA-approved levalbuterol is available for administration to this patient receiving mechanical ventilation?

2. What is the amount of FDA-approved levalbuterol available by these formulations?

3. The respiratory therapist consults with the pulmonologists concerning the levalbuterol treatments being delivered via pMDI. The physician would like levalbuterol to be administered using an SVN. The ventilator does not have a nebulizer function to power the nebulizer, so the therapist is considering using an externally powered gas source (wall flow meter) to power the nebulizer. Are there any problems that you would want to discuss with the physician with the use of this method of nebulization?

4. The physician still wants a nebulizer to be used for the administration of albuterol. Is another option available for nebulization of medications?

5. The therapist gives this option to the doctor, and the doctor asks: "What about taking the patient off the ventilator and manually ventilating during aerosol administration?" What should be the therapist's response to this question?

6. The doctor finally agrees with your suggestion for nebulizing albuterol. Now the doctor's concern is where the nebulizer should be placed to obtain the greatest deposition of medication. What should the therapist recommend?

18 Skeletal Muscle Relaxants (Neuromuscular Blocking Agents)

CHAPTER OUTLINE

CHAPTER OBJECTIVES

After answering the following questions, the reader should be able to:

1. Define terms that pertain to skeletal muscle relaxants
2. Define neuromuscular blocking agents (NMBAs)
3. List the uses of NMBAs
4. Describe physiology of the neuromuscular junction
5. Describe the makeup of nondepolarizing agents
6. Describe the makeup of depolarizing agents
7. Describe uses of NMBAs and mechanical ventilation
8. Identify methods of monitoring neuromuscular blockade

KEY TERMS AND DEFINITIONS

Match the following definitions with their terms.

1. _____ This is the accidental inhalation of food particles, fluids, or gastric contents into the lungs.

2. _____ One of the basic functional units of the nervous system that is specialized to transmit electrical nerve impulses and carry information from one part of the body to another; it consists of a cell body, axons, and dendrites.

3. _____ Pneumonia that is acquired in a health care setting.

4. _____ A chemical that is released from a nerve ending to transmit an impulse from a nerve cell to another nerve, muscle, organ, or other tissue.

5. _____ Characteristics of a substance or drug with the ability to cause total or partial loss of memory.

6. _____ Involuntary contractions or twitching of groups of muscle fibers.

a. Acetylcholinesterase (AchE)
b. Amnestic properties
c. Aspiration
d. Fasciculations
e. Myasthenia gravis
f. Neuromuscular blocking agent (NMBA)
g. Neuron (nerve cell)
h. Neurotransmitter
i. Nosocomial pneumonia
j. Sedation
k. Status asthmaticus
l. Status epilepticus
m. Receptor
n. Somatic motor neurons

7. _____ An enzyme that breaks down the neurotransmitter acetylcholine at the synaptic cleft, so that the next nerve impulse can be transmitted across the synaptic gap.

8. _____ The production of a restful state of mind, particularly by the use of drugs that have a calming effect, relieving anxiety and tension.

9. _____ An autoimmune neuromuscular disorder characterized by chronic fatigue and exhaustion of muscles.

10. _____ A person having at least 30 minutes of continuous seizure activity without full recovery between seizures.

11. _____ A substance that interferes with the neural transmission between motor neurons and skeletal muscles.

12. _____ An attack of asthma lasting for more than 24 hours.

13. _____ A molecular structure inside or outside the cell that binds to a specific substance to elicit a physiologic response.

14. _____ is part of the nervous system that controls muscles that arc under voluntary control.

USES OF NEUROMUSCULAR BLOCKING AGENTS

15. Explain the difference between the mechanism of action for depolarizing and nondepolarizing agents.

16. Name a depolarizing drug currently available.

17. List eight clinical uses of NMBAs.

   a. _____

   b. _____

   c. _____

   d. _____

   e. _____

   f. _____

   g. _____

   h. _____

18. What is the most common pathologic condition requiring a patient to be placed on mechanical ventilation and require muscle relaxation?

Chapter **18 Skeletal Muscle Relaxants (Neuromuscular Blocking Agents)**

PHYSIOLOGY OF THE NEUROMUSCULAR JUNCTION

19. The somatic motor nervous system, or skeletal muscle system, controls what type of movement?

20. What is considered the major muscle of ventilation?

21. The autonomic nervous system controls what type of movement?

22. The transmission of nerve conduction in skeletal muscle is chemically mediated by what neurotransmitter?

23. Acetylcholine is then broken down and inactivated by the enzyme _____, allowing the muscle fiber to repolarize.

24. Based on neuromuscular physiology, describe two ways muscle contraction may be blocked.

   a. _____

   b. _____

NONDEPOLARIZING AGENTS

25. Where do nondepolarizing agents cause muscle paralysis by affecting the postsynaptic cholinergic receptors?

26. Give an example of a cholinesterase inhibitor that can reverse nondepolarizing agents.

27. Nondepolarizing agents have a longer duration of action than the depolarizing agent _____.

28. What medication has the greatest potential to cause cardiovascular side effects, especially tachycardia and hypertension?

29. What are two concerns to respiratory therapists when administering nondepolarizing agents?

   a. _____

   b. _____

30. Which reversal agent is used to treat myasthenia gravis?

31. What drug is used to reverse succinylcholine?

32. Explain the term *Hofmann degradation* as it relates to elimination of atracurium and cistracurium.

33. What two NMBAs would not be recommended for a patient with high blood pressure and tachycardia?

   a. _____

   b. _____

34. List two side effects of reversing agents.

   a. _____

   b. _____

DEPOLARIZING AGENTS

35. List the only depolarizing agent available in the United States and its main indication for use.

36. Fill in the chart below.

Depolarizing Agent	Intravenous (IV) Dose	Time to Total Muscle Paralysis (seconds)	Clinical Duration (minutes)

37. List seven adverse effects of succinylcholine that can occur in adult patients:

    a. _____

    b. _____

    c. _____

    d. _____

    e. _____

    f. _____

    g. _____

NEUROMUSCULAR BLOCKING AGENTS AND MECHANICAL VENTILATION

38. List six disease states in which neuromuscular blockade may be beneficial.

    a. _____

    b. _____

    c. _____

    d. _____

    e. _____

    f. _____

39. In paralyzed patients receiving mechanical ventilation, elevating the head may reduce the risk of _____.

40. It is important to remember that NMBAs only cause muscle paralysis. What should be administered to remove conscious awareness and to provide pain relief?

41. What agents are preferred for paralysis of ventilated patients because of the predictability, longer duration of action, and manageable side effects of these agents?

     Chapter **18** Skeletal Muscle Relaxants (Neuromuscular Blocking Agents)

MONITORING OF NEUROMUSCULAR BLOCKADE

42. List five clinical factors that can potentiate the effects of neuromuscular blockade.

    a. _____

    b. _____

    c. _____

    d. _____

    e. _____

43. List two clinical factors that can inhibit the effects of neuromuscular blockade.

    a. _____

    b. _____

44. List, in order of occurrence, the sequence of paralysis of the skeletal muscles that can be monitored physically.

    1. _____

    2. _____

    3. _____

    4. _____

    5. _____

    6. _____

    7. _____

45. During brief periods of paralysis, two simple measures of voluntary muscular function include subjective assessments such as:

    a. _____

    b. _____

46. If you were able to develop the perfect NMBA, what characteristics would it possess?

NATIONAL BOARD OF RESPIRATORY CARE (NBRC) TESTING QUESTIONS

1. Which of the following are indications for administration of an NMBA?
   1. Endotracheal extubation
   2. Muscle paralysis during surgery
   3. To facilitate mechanical ventilation
   4. Endotracheal intubation
      a. 1 and 2 only
      b. 3 and 4 only
      c. 2, 3, and 4 only
      d. 1, 2, and 3 only

2. If a mechanically ventilated patient is receiving vecuronium, the patient should also receive which of the following?
    1. Sedation
    2. Analgesics
    3. Frequent suctioning
    4. Bronchodilator therapy
        a. 1 and 2 only
        b. 3 and 4 only
        c. 2, 3, and 4 only
        d. 1, 2, and 4 only

3. Which of the following best defines an NMBA?
    a. Drugs that partially block selected skeletal muscles, such as the diaphragm
    b. Drugs that reduce heart rate and blood pressure during invasive medical procedures
    c. Drugs that minimize brain activity for traumatic brain injury
    d. Drugs that paralyze muscles and prevent movement

4. Which of the following is considered a depolarizing NMBA?
    a. Vecuronium
    b. Rocuronium
    c. Pancuronium
    d. Succinylcholine

5. Muscle paralysis caused by nondepolarizing blocking agents can be reversed using which of the following?
    a. Cholinesterase
    b. Cholinesterase inhibitors
    c. Parasympatholytics
    d. Sympathomimetics

6. The transmission of nerve conduction in skeletal muscle is chemically mediated by which neurotransmitter?
    a. Acetylcholine
    b. Serotonin
    c. Acetylcholinesterase
    d. Norepinephrine

7. Which of the following drugs can reverse the effects of nondepolarizing blockade?
    1. Edrophonium
    2. Pyridostigmine
    3. Neostigmine
    4. Rocuronium
        a. 1 and 2 only
        b. 1, 2, and 3 only
        c. 2, 3, and 4 only
        d. 1, 2, 3, and 4

8. A cardiac patient requires intubation and mechanical ventilation. Which of the following NMBAs should be administered to minimize any potential for cardiac side effects?
    a. Vecuronium
    b. Atropine
    c. Pancuronium
    d. Succinylcholine

9. The neuromuscular drug of choice to assist in endotracheal intubation is:
    a. Vecuronium
    b. Atracurium
    c. Mivacurium
    d. Succinylcholine

10. For endotracheally intubated, paralyzed patients receiving mechanical ventilation, which of the following may help reduce the risk of aspiration?
    a. Reduce the ventilator driving pressure
    b. Elevate the head of the bed
    c. Have the patient supine with legs raised
    d. Reduce the positive end-expiratory pressure (PEEP) to less than 5 cm H_2O.

11. What is the intravenous dose for succinylcholine?
    a. 0.3-1.0 mg/kg
    b. 0.5-0.8 mg/kg
    c. 1.0-1.5 mg/kg
    d. 2.0-2.5 mg/kg

12. What is the simplest way to monitor the adequacy of neuromuscular blockade?
    a. Train of four
    b. Twitch monitoring
    c. Response to painful stimuli
    d. Direct observation of muscle activity

13. What would likely be the first indication that a nondepolarizing agent is reversing?
    a. Eyelids move, and the eyes move back and forth.
    b. Extremities move with twitching and spasms.
    c. The diaphragm contracts, indicated by abdominal wall movement.
    d. The patient swallows and coughs.

14. During brief periods of paralysis, which of the following subjective assessments measure voluntary muscular functions?
    1. Hand grip strength
    2. The ability to lift the head off the bed for 5 seconds
    3. Heart rate returning to normal
    4. Increase in SpO_2
        a. 1 and 2 only
        b. 2 and 3 only
        c. 1, 3, and 4 only
        d. 1, 2, and 4 only

15. Repolarization of the muscle fiber occurs when acetylcholine is broken down and inactivated by the enzyme:
    a. Acetylcholinesterase
    b. Neostigmine
    c. Cholinesterase
    d. Acetylcholine

16. Nondepolarizing agents cause muscle paralysis by affecting the postsynaptic cholinergic receptors at the:
    a. Synaptic cleft
    b. Neuromuscular junction
    c. Dendrite
    d. Neuroeffector site

17. When a nondepolarizing agent is administered in a nonintubated patient, what should the respiratory therapist be concerned with?
    1. The intracranial pressures
    2. Maintaining a patent airway
    3. The appropriate size suction catheter to be used
    4. Maintaining appropriate ventilation
        a. 2 and 4 only
        b. 1 and 3 only
        c. 1, 2, and 4 only
        d. 2, 3, and 4 only

160

18. To reduce the adverse effects of NMBAs, which of the following medications can be given?
    a. Atropine
    b. Neostigmine
    c. Edrophonium
    d. Quafenisine

19. Which of the following indicates initial depolarization after administration of succinylcholine?
    a. Tachycardia
    b. Hypertension
    c. Fasciculations
    d. Paralysis

20. Which of the following NMBAs cannot be reversed with medication?
    a. Pancuronium
    b. Succinylcholine
    c. Rocuronium
    d. Vecuronium

CASE STUDY 1

You are called to the emergency department to assist in the care of patient who was in a motor vehicle accident. In the report, you learn that he has pulmonary contusions and a flail chest. He is not responding to verbal commands and is combative. On the basis of his arterial blood gases and other physical findings, you recommend that the patient be orally intubated.

1. Which NMBA would you use to paralyze him? Why?

The patient is intubated and moved to the intensive care unit, where he is placed on mechanical ventilation. Over the next few hours, the patient remains very restless. He is breathing asynchronously with the ventilator in spite of several changes made to the ventilator settings. Physical assessment reveals:
    Respiratory rate: 30 breaths/min
    Blood pressure: 170/100 mm Hg
    Pulse: 148 beats/min
    You call the physician and suggest an NMBA.

2. Which classification of NMBA would you recommend?

3. Based on the patient's physical assessment, what agents would be most appropriate to use? Why?

4. What type of blocking agent would you *not* want to use for this patient, and why?

Chapter **18 Skeletal Muscle Relaxants (Neuromuscular Blocking Agents)**

5. Are there any other medications you would suggest for this patient receiving NMBAs?

The patient has been given an NMBA, is now paralyzed, and has received a sedative and pain medication.

6. How could you determine that the patient received an appropriate amount of medication to reduce pain and anxiety adequately?

7. Because clinical signs are lost with paralysis, what should be monitored continuously to assess signs of restlessness, anxiety, and distress?

CASE STUDY 2

A patient diagnosed with severe asthma exacerbation has been intubated and is receiving pressure-controlled ventilation. Despite numerous changes to the ventilator settings, the patient is agitated and is "fighting the ventilator," according to the respiratory therapist. The respiratory therapist has decided to call the pulmonologist for an order for an NMBA.

1. What would be a clinical indication for administration of an NMBA for this patient?

2. Which classification of NMBAs would you suggest for this patient?

3. If the physician were to ask for your recommendation about an NMBA for this patient, what agent would be least appropriate to administer? What would be the best agent to administer?

The patient is now paralyzed and is breathing synchronously with the ventilator.

4. While the patient is intubated and receiving mechanical ventilation, what can you do to reduce the incidence of nosocomial infection and aspiration while the patient is receiving an NMBA?

The next day it is decided to begin reversing the NMBA.

5. What would be a quick, subjective assessment to determine the depth of blockade and voluntary muscle function?

6. What could you use to assess the patient's muscle strength objectively?

The physician has now administered a reversing agent.

7. What would be the first response indicating the patient has begun breathing on his own?

Chapter **18 Skeletal Muscle Relaxants (Neuromuscular Blocking Agents)**

19 Diuretic Agents

CHAPTER OUTLINE

Key Terms and Definitions
Renal Structure and Function
Diuretic Groups
Diuretics and Acute Respiratory Distress Syndrome
National Board of Respiratory Care (NBRC) Testing Questions
Case Studies 1 and 2

CHAPTER OBJECTIVES

After answering the following questions, the reader should be able to:

1. Define terms pertaining to diuretic agents
2. Describe renal function, filtration, reabsorption, and acid–base balance
3. List and describe the various groups of diuretics
4. List some of the indications for diuretic therapy
5. List the most common adverse reactions associated with the use of diuretics
6. Describe special situations related to diuretic therapy

KEY TERMS AND DEFINITIONS

Match the following definitions with their terms.

1. _____ Swelling resulting from an abnormal accumulation of fluid in intercellular spaces of the body.

2. _____ Abnormally decreased volume of blood circulating in the body.

3. _____ The microscopic functional unit of the kidney responsible for filtering and maintaining fluid balance; each kidney is made of approximately 2 million of these.

4. _____ Inadequacy of the heart as a pump, failing to maintain adequacy of blood circulation, with resulting congestion and tissue edema.

5. _____ Amount of urine produced in 24 hours; normal urine output averages 30-60 mL/hour.

6. _____ The return to the blood of most of the water, sodium (Na^+), amino acids, and sugar that were removed during filtration; occurs mainly in the proximal tubule of the nephron.

7. _____ The mechanism by which the hydrostatic pressure forces fluid out of the glomerular capillary into the renal ducts.

a. Congestive heart failure (CHF)
b. Edema
c. Glomerular filtration
d. Hypovolemia
e. Nephrocalcinosis
f. Nephron
g. Ototoxicity
h. Reabsorption
i. Synergistic effect
j. Urine output
k. Diuretic

8. _____ Renal lithiasis in which calcium deposits form in the renal parenchyma and result in reduced kidney function and the presence of blood in the urine.

9. _____ Damage to the ear, specifically the cochlea or auditory nerve and sometimes the vestibulum, by a toxin.

10. _____ Situation in which the effect of two chemicals on an organism is greater than the effect of each chemical individually.

11. _____ A drug that increases urine output.

RENAL STRUCTURE AND FUNCTION

12. List the three basic functions of the renal system.

   a. _____

   b. _____

   c. _____

13. From which artery does the kidney receive blood flow?

14. What is the name of the hormone produced by the posterior pituitary gland that aids in the regulation of urine output?

15. From where is aldosterone secreted?

16. Explain how an increase in a patient's preload can result in an increased urine output.

17. What will force Na^+ exchange for H^+, thereby producing metabolic alkalosis?

18. Most filtered K^+ is reabsorbed in the proximal tubules. Where is the K^+ found in the urine is that secreted?

19. Where are chloride and bicarbonate are passively reabsorbed?

DIURETIC GROUPS

20. What is the main purpose of diuretics?

21. How do most diuretics work?

22. List one of the most common uses of osmotic diuretics.

23. Osmotic substances are potent diuretics that lead to increased excretion of _____ and _____.

24. List three common uses for carbonic anhydrase inhibitors (CAIs).

    a. _____

    b. _____

    c. _____

25. Explain the mechanism of action for loop diuretics.

26. When loop diuretics are administered to patients with pulmonary edema what happens?

27. Apart from their diuretic effects, loop diuretics may cause what type of acute effect?

28. How long after administration of a loop diuretic should diuresis take place? What would you suggest to the physician if it does not happen?

29. What is the mechanism of action for thiazide diuretics? Why are they not as potent as other diuretics?

30. List a clinical indication for the administration of thiazide diuretics.

31. Explain the mechanism of action for K^+-sparing diuretics.

32. What is the most common diuretic combination?

33. List three major complications or adverse effects of diuretics.

a. _____

b. _____

c. _____

34. List three indications for K$^+$ supplementation.

a. _____

b. _____

c. _____

35. What is the term used to describe an increased blood glucose level, associated with the use of loop and thiazide diuretics?

36. One of the least toxic and most effective loop diuretics in pediatric practice is _____.

DIURETICS AND ACUTE RESPIRATORY DISTRESS SYNDROME

37. According to the Fluid and Catheter Treatment Trial (FACTT), what three positive outcomes were the result of conservative fluid management for acute respiratory distress syndrome (ARDS)?

a. _____

b. _____

c. _____

38. Fill in the following table regarding the class, mechanism of action, main indication, and other uses of diuretics.

Diuretic Class (Mechanism of Action)	Main Indications	Other Uses
Osmotic Diuretics		
Carbonic Anhydrase Inhibitors		
Loop Diuretics		
Thiazide Diuretics		

Diuretic Class (Mechanism of Action)	Main Indications	Other Uses
K^+-Sparing Diuretics		

NATIONAL BOARD OF RESPIRATORY CARE (NBRC) TESTING QUESTIONS

1. Urine output less than 30 to 60 mL/hour is known as _____.
   a. Polyuria
   b. Anuria
   c. Oliguria
   d. Nephronemia

2. Carbonic anhydrase inhibitors act in which of the following?
   a. Proximal tubules
   b. Distal tubules
   c. Loop of Henle
   d. Glomerulus

3. Approximately what percentage of the cardiac output in a normal 70-kg adult flows through the kidneys?
   a. 10
   b. 15
   c. 20
   d. 22

4. Potassium-sparing diuretics interfere with the sodium/potassium exchange in the:
   a. Distal convulated tubule
   b. Loop of Henle
   c. Proximal tubule
   d. Bladder

5. Normal urine output averages:
   a. 10 to 30 mL/hour
   b. 30 to 60 mL/hour
   c. 100 to 120 mL/hour
   d. 120 to 140 mL/hour

6. Which of the following is the most common combination of diuretics?
   a. Mannitol and thiazide
   b. Loop and carbonic anhydrase inhibitor
   c. Thiazide and carbonic anhydrase inhibitor
   d. Loop and thiazide

7. The functional unit of the kidneys is called the:
   a. Ureter
   b. Nephron
   c. Urethra
   d. Loop of Henle

8. The K^+ found in the urine is that secreted by which of the following?
   a. Distal tubule
   b. Proximal tubule
   c. Nephrons
   d. Central tubules

9. Osmotic diuretics are potent diuretics that lead to increased excretion of which of the following?
   a. Magnesium
   b. Glucose and water
   c. Water and NaCl
   d. Sodium

10. If a patient has hypokalemia, which of the following acid–base disturbances is most likely?
    a. Respiratory acidosis
    b. Metabolic alkalosis
    c. Respiratory alkalosis
    d. Metabolic acidosis

11. The drug of choice to treat cerebral edema is:
    a. Furosemide
    b. Diamox
    c. Mannitol
    d. Benzthiazide

12. Patients receiving loop diuretics should have _____ levels monitored.
    a. Bicarbonate
    b. pH
    c. Bleeding time
    d. Electrolytes

13. A patient receiving loop diuretics should experience diuresis within:
    a. 1 hour
    b. 20 minutes
    c. 2 hours
    d. 24 hours

14. The main reason for administering a loop diuretic to a patient with pulmonary edema is:
    a. To reduce inflammation in the airways
    b. To cause pulmonary artery vasoconstriction and reduce pulmonary vascular resistance
    c. To increase left heart pressure
    d. To cause diuresis and reduce pulmonary edema

15. For pediatric patients, the least toxic and most effective diuretic is:
    a. Mannitol
    b. CAI
    c. Furosemide
    d. Isosorbide

16. Within 5 minutes of the administration of intravenous loop diuretics to cardiac patients, which of the following effects is observed?
    a. Vasoconstriction
    b. Vasodilation
    c. Edema
    d. Hypertonicity

17. Osmotic diuretics are often used in the management of which of the following?
    a. Traumatic brain injury
    b. Kidney failure
    c. Ascites
    d. Liver failure

18. Thiazide diuretics are considered to be first line of therapy for which of the following?
    a. Left heart failure
    b. Cor pulmonale
    c. Mild hypertension
    d. Acute renal failure

19. Which of the following are the most common side effects of diuretic therapy?
    1. Hypervolemia
    2. Hypovolemia
    3. Reduced cerebral perfusion
    4. Acid–base abnormalities
        a. 1 and 3 only
        b. 2 and 4 only
        c. 2, 3, and 4 only
        d. 1, 3, and 4 only

20. Although CAIs are considered to be very weak diuretics, they are commonly used to treat which of the following?
    1. Glaucoma
    2. Metabolic alkalosis
    3. Motion sickness
    4. Altitude sickness
        a. 1 and 2 only
        b. 1, 2, and 3 only
        c. 2, 3, and 4 only
        d. 1, 2, and 4 only

CASE STUDY 1

Mrs. S. has been brought to the emergency department (ED) with chief complaints of increasing shortness of breath, coughing, and mild substernal pressure. Her husband called the paramedics when she complained she "cannot breathe." Mrs. S. is currently on a Venturi mask with an inspired oxygen fraction (Fio_2) of 0.50. Her husband states she is a 66-year-old housewife with a history of coronary artery disease, arrhythmia, and a recent hospitalization for 3 weeks, resulting from an anterior wall myocardial infarction (MI); she has been out of the hospital for a month. Physical examination reveals a heart rate of 158 beats/min, blood pressure of 110/70 mm Hg, and a Spo_2 of 93% on the Venturi mask. Breath sounds reveal inspiratory crackles from the bases up to the midchest, with mild expiratory wheezes. Her respiratory rate is 34 breaths/min, with some paradoxical respirations noted. Pitting edema is present in the ankles, no clubbing or cyanosis is noted, and her skin is cool and diaphoretic. There is jugular vein distention noted.

Mrs. S. has been admitted to the cardiac care unit. A portable chest radiograph taken on admission in the ED has now been returned and reveals cardiomegaly, as well as bilateral pulmonary vascular engorgement with interstitial and alveolar edema. She is diagnosed with congestive heart failure.

1. What drug would be beneficial in helping remove fluid from the patient's lungs?

2. Thirty minutes after giving 40 mg of Lasix, diuresis has not occurred. What would you now recommend?

It has been 2 hours since Mrs. S. was admitted to the cardiac care unit. She is resting more comfortably and is on a nasal cannula at 3 L/minute. Because of the medications she is currently receiving, laboratory tests are obtained with the following results:

Potassium: 2.5 mEq/L (normal: 3.5-5.0 mEq/L)
Sodium: 140 mEq/L (normal: 136-145 mEq/L)
Chloride: 87 mEq/L (normal: 95-105 mEq/L)
Glucose: 125 mg/dL (normal: 90-150 mg/dL)

3. On the basis of this finding, what would you recommend?

4. What acid–base imbalance is likely to occur with these chemistry results?

You are the day shift supervisor for a 300-bed hospital in the respiratory therapy department. You are making rounds in the morning when your beeper alerts you to come to the ED.

A patient has been admitted with severe headache. Blood pressure is 160/100 mm Hg, pulse is 128 beats/min, and respirations are 26 breaths/min. Chest radiograph reveals a normal-size heart, and the lungs are normal. After administering oxygen to the patient, it has been decided to administer a diuretic.

1. Which diuretic class would be best for this patient?

2. Explain the action of this diuretic.

You are now called to the intensive care unit, where a patient has been admitted after a motorcycle accident. The patient has sustained a head injury. Computed tomography scan shows contusions and brain swelling. The patient has been placed on mechanical ventilation.

3. Which diuretic class would be indicated for this patient?

4. Explain the action of this diuretic.

This patient has now been stabilized, and you are paged to the ED. On entering the ED, you are informed that a 75-year-old man has complaints of severe eye pain, nausea, and vomiting. The patient's eyes are red, and he complains of blurred vision.

5. What diuretic class would be most helpful for this patient's condition?

6. Explain the action of this diuretic.

20 Drugs Affecting the Central Nervous System

CHAPTER OBJECTIVES

After answering the following questions, the reader should be able to:

1. Define key terms pertaining to drugs that affect the central nervous system (CNS)
2. Describe the multiple functions of the CNS
3. Recognize various effects of medications on the CNS and their abilities to modulate neurotransmitters
4. Comprehend psychiatric medications, including classification, use, and side effect profiles
5. Recognize the effects of alcohol on the CNS during acute intoxication, chronic use, and after abrupt withdrawal
6. Distinguish physiologic and psychological bases of pain and the classes of analgesics used to treat pain
7. Recognize indications for the use of both local and general anesthesia
8. Describe the concept of conscious sedation and indications and guidelines for use
9. Distinguish drugs that stimulate the CNS and respiratory system and describe the indications for application

KEY TERMS AND DEFINITIONS

Match the following definitions with their terms.

1. _____ The brain and spinal cord make up the functional components of this system; together these provide for all conscious and subconscious functions of the body.

2. _____ These drugs can alter levels of certain neurotransmitters, in particular norepinephrine and serotonin within the brain.

    a. Analgesics
    b. Anesthetics
    c. Antidepressants
    d. Antipsychotics
    e. Anxiolytics
    f. Central nervous system (CNS)
    g. Cholinesterase inhibitors

3. _____ These drugs depress the nervous system; they can be divided into two categories, local and general. Their use results in the absence of pain perception.

4. _____ These drugs are used primarily to treat bipolar disorders.

5. _____ These drugs provide pain relief; they can be subdivided into narcotic and nonnarcotic medications.

6. _____ These drugs are used to treat psychotic disorders, such as schizophrenia, and they affect primarily the neurotransmitter dopamine.

7. _____ This is a method used during certain invasive procedures; the goals of this method are to decrease the level of consciousness and relieve anxiety and pain, while allowing the patient to follow verbal commands.

8. _____ These drugs can cause increased activity of the brain.

9. _____ These drugs are known as minor tranquilizers; they treat several conditions, including anxiety disorders and insomnia.

10. _____ These drugs block the activity of cholinesterase, an enzyme that inactivates the neurotransmitter acetylcholine.

11. _____ This is a chemical substance that allows neurons to transmit electrical impulses throughout the CNS and peripheral nervous system.

h. Conscious sedation
i. Mood stabilizers
j. Neurotransmitter
k. Stimulants

BRAIN STRUCTURE AND FUNCTION

12. Give a brief description of the following areas of the brain.
    a. Cortex
    b. Midbrain
    c. Brainstem or medulla

13. What disease is caused by a loss of neurons containing dopamine in the midbrain and is characterized by resting tremor and gait disturbances?

NEUROTRANSMITTERS

14. The clinical effects of CNS drugs depend on what factor?

15. Do CNS drugs increase or decrease individual neuronal activity?

16. The effect of the neurotransmitter released is determined by what six factors?

    a. _____

    b. _____

    c. _____

    d. _____

    e. _____

    f. _____

PSYCHIATRIC MEDICATIONS

Antidepressants

17. Deficiency of what two neurotransmitters has been linked to depression?

18. List three etiologies of depressive disorders.

    a. _____

    b. _____

    c. _____

19. Fill in the drug class and U.S. brand names for the following drugs used to treat depression.

Class	Generic Drug	Brand Name
	Citalopram	
	Fluoxetine	
	Olanzapine and Fluoxetine	
	Fluvoxamine Maleate	
	Paroxetine	
	Sertraline	
	Escitalopram oxalate	
	Venlafaxine	
	Duloxetine	
	Desvenlafaxine	
	Nefazodone	
	Bupropion	
	Bupropion and Naltrexone	

Class	Generic Drug	Brand Name
	Amitriptyline	
	Amoxapine	
	Clomipramine	
	Desipramine	
	Doxepin	
	Imipramine	
	Nortriptyline	
	Protriptyline	
	Trimipramine	
	Mirtazapine	
	Phenelzine	
	Tranylcypromine	
	Isocarboxazid	
	St. John's wort *(Hypericum perforatum)*	

Mood Stabilizers

20. Pharmacologic treatment of bipolar disorder typically begins with what type of medications?

21. Define bipolar disorder.

Antipsychotics

22. What neurotransmitter does pharmacotherapy for psychosis associated with depression or mania generally aim to increase?

Drugs for Alzheimer's Dementia: Cholinesterase Inhibitors

23. Deficits of which neurotransmitter are associated with cognitive deficits in patients with Alzheimer's dementia?

24. What type of drug can improve cognition and function in patients with Alzheimer's disease?

Anxiolytics

25. List the drugs that are used to treat anxiety and insomnia.

26. When given with opioids, what side effect could benzodiazepines augment?

Barbiturates and Other Hypnotics

27. When choosing a sedative drug for your patient, why would you choose a benzodiazepine over a barbiturate?

28. For the following drugs, give an indication for each of them.

    a. Thiopental: _____

    b. Pentobarbital: _____

    c. Phenobarbital: _____

29. What is a common complaint that frequently results in the prescription of a hypnotic?

ETHYL ALCOHOL

30. What is considered a toxic level of blood alcohol? What side effect from toxic levels would concern you?

31. What can the abrupt withdrawal after prolonged use of alcohol cause?

32. True or False: Alcohol is metabolized to carbon dioxide (CO_2) and water (H_2O) and produces acetaldehyde in the process.

PAIN TREATMENT

33. What is pain?

34. What are two components of the pain experience?

    a._____

    b. _____

35. How do nonsteroidal anti-inflammatory drugs (NSAIDs) work?

36. What is the most frequently used analgesic?

37. Your patient was just brought into the emergency department (ED) in respiratory arrest after taking hydromorphone while his Duragesic patch was on. What medication would you give to reverse his respiratory depression?

38. List a reason for allowing patients to use a patient-controlled analgesia (PCA) device to control their pain.

39. Depth of anesthesia is determined by the patient's response to painful stimuli and is often judged by the changes in what two sympathetic responses?

Conscious Sedation

40. During conscious sedation, patients should remain _____ and able to communicate, protect their own _____, and breathe adequately.

41. How many qualified people must be continuously present during the sedation period?

42. Because of the potential for airway compromise, what should the respiratory therapist have available to maintain a patent airway?

43. What recommendations for monitoring are suggested during conscious sedation?

    a. _____

    b. _____

    c. _____

    d. _____

CENTRAL NERVOUS SYSTEM AND RESPIRATORY STIMULANTS

44. What is a common component in popular beverages and is used therapeutically in apnea-bradycardia syndromes of premature births?

NATIONAL BOARD OF RESPIRATORY CARE (NBRC) TESTING QUESTIONS

1. The area of the brain that controls motor function and coordinates movement is the:
   a. Cerebrum
   b. Diencephalon
   c. Brainstem
   d. Cerebellum

2. Control of breathing is regulated mainly in the:
   a. Cerebrum
   b. Diencephalon
   c. Brainstem
   d. Cerebellum

3. Psychotic disorders are characterized by:
   a. Unstable gait
   b. Rigidity and hypertonicity
   c. Excessive fidgeting
   d. Impaired reality testing

4. Which of the following is considered to be a toxic level of alcohol?
   a. 200 to 300 mg/dL
   b. 325 to 400 mg/dL
   c. 425 to 500 mg/dL
   d. 400 to 600 mg/dL

5. Which class of analgesics may enhance bronchodilation and suppress cough when administered by inhalation?
   a. Alcohol
   b. NSAIDs
   c. Local anesthetics
   d. Barbiturates

6. A disease characterized by resting tremor, rigidity, and postural instability resulting from loss of dopamine-containing neurons is:
   a. Parkinson's disease
   b. Delirium tremens
   c. Manic depression
   d. Bipolar disorder

7. These drugs, subdivided into narcotic and nonnarcotic medications, provide pain relief:
   a. Anxiolytics
   b. Mood stabilizers
   c. Analgesics
   d. Cholinesterase inhibitors

8. The brain is composed of which of the following?
   1. Cortex
   2. Spinal cord
   3. Brainstem
   4. Midbrain
      a. 1 and 2 only
      b. 3 and 4 only
      c. 2, 3, and 4 only
      d. 1, 3, and 4 only

9. Medical treatment of any degree of bipolar disorder must begin with which of the following medications?
   a. Opioid analgesic
   b. Mood stabilizer
   c. Barbiturates
   d. Antidepressants

10. A person diagnosed with Alzheimer's disease would have improvement of cognition and function with the use of this class of drugs:
    a. Mood stabilizers
    b. Sympathomimetics
    c. Cholinesterase inhibitors
    d. Pain relievers

11. Which of the following drugs is recommended to control seizures?
    a. Thiopental
    b. Pentobarbital
    c. Norepinephrine
    d. Phenobarbital

12. As alcohol is broken down and metabolized into CO_2 and H_2O, the by-product is:
    a. Acetaldehyde
    b. Dopamine
    c. Norepinephrine
    d. Acetylcysteine

13. Chronic pain can be controlled by antidepressants and _____.
    a. Mood stabilizers
    b. Analgesics
    c. Tranquilizers
    d. Anesthetics

14. The most frequently used analgesic NSAID that can be purchased over the counter is:
    a. Lithium
    b. Ethanol
    c. Aspirin
    d. Phenobarbital

15. Depth of anesthesia is determined by the patient's response to painful stimuli and is often judged by the sympathetic response, which is:
    a. Twitching of the extremities
    b. Lack of feeling in the extremities
    c. A change in heart rate or blood pressure
    d. A drop in arterial oxygen saturation

16. Which of the following procedures has guidelines requiring that at least the operator and a monitoring assistant must be present during administration?
    a. General anesthesia
    b. Conscious sedation
    c. Intravenous opioids
    d. Local anesthesia

17. Respiratory failure resulting from sedative or opioid drug overdose can be treated with which of the following specific antagonists?
    a. Methylxanthines
    b. Morphine
    c. Naloxone
    d. Caffeine

18. A hospitalized patient is complaining of insomnia and anxiety related to upcoming procedures. A drug that would help treat these conditions would be which of the following?
    a. Haldol
    b. Lithium
    c. Xanax
    d. Prozac

19. What is considered to be the fifth vital sign?
    a. Oxygen saturation
    b. Pain
    c. Eye movement
    d. Finger movement

20. A patient has continual complaints of pain. When asked how intense the pain is, the patient keeps saying: "It hurts." Which of the following would be a way to have the patient estimate the magnitude of the pain?
    a. Have the patient point to the painful area.
    b. Have the patient describe in detail the pain.
    c. Have the patient relate a past painful experience to this one.
    d. Use a numeric analog pain scale.

You are the day-shift respiratory therapy supervisor, and you will be involved in treating various patients throughout the day. Your responsibilities today will take you to the ED, the intensive care unit (ICU), labor and delivery, and the neonatal ICU. Your task, if you decide to take it, will be to assist in decision-making opportunities in treating these patients. Good luck.

You are called to the ED, where you find Mr. Jones, a 67-year-old patient with chronic obstructive pulmonary disease (COPD) who has been admitted with pneumonia. His respiratory rate is 34 breaths/min, he has prolonged exhalation and accessory muscle usage, and he is breathing with a 2-L/min nasal cannula. His arterial blood gas (ABG) shows the following: pH, 7.21; partial pressure of arterial carbon dioxide ($Paco_2$), 74 mm Hg; partial pressure of arterial oxygen (Pao_2), 49 mm Hg; bicarbonate (HCO_3), 34 mEq/L. The resident wants to give a respiratory stimulant, an analeptic drug, to stimulate his breathing to "blow off" the CO_2. You enter the patient's room just as the resident is asking the nurse to give the drug.

1. What would you recommend?

You are now called by a nurse on the floors. The nurse tells you that a patient is about to go home, and this patient would like her respiratory treatment before she leaves. After the treatment, the patient asks what you would recommend for a medication to help with her pain. She explains that the pain is getting better, but she still has mild pain and she does not want a prescription.

2. What medication would you suggest?

After leaving this patient, you are paged to labor and delivery, where a 32-week gestational age infant is born via cesarean section. The mother received several drugs, one of which was an opioid. The infant is not responding to typical stimuli and is currently being hand ventilated with a resuscitation bag.

3. What drug should be given to reverse the effects of the opioid?

From here you are called to neonatal ICU. The respiratory therapist is about to implement continuous positive airway pressure (CPAP) therapy on a 27-week infant who had been receiving mechanical ventilation. The therapist has reported to you that the infant has had some episodes of apnea, and the therapist is concerned about placing the infant on CPAP. The therapist asks you to recommend a drug that would stimulate the infant's breathing.

4. What would you recommend?

A patient in the ICU is about to have a medical procedure performed at the bedside. After the patient has signed the consent form, she asks what comfort measures will be administered during the procedure. You tell her that she will be receiving conscious sedation. She does not understand what this means.

1. How would you explain what conscious sedation is and how it will make her more comfortable during the procedure?

2. In preparation for the procedure, what should the respiratory therapist have available to maintain the patient's airway?

3. The patient would like to know who else will be in the room besides the respiratory therapist and how she will be monitored. What would you tell this patient?

4. As you are preparing the resuscitation equipment, the patient's nurse tells you that she has never assisted in conscious sedation. She would like to know how many people need to be present during the sedation period. What would you tell the nurse?

21 Vasopressors, Inotropes, and Antiarrhythmic Agents

CHAPTER OUTLINE

CHAPTER OBJECTIVES

After answering the following questions, the reader should be able to:

1. Define terms that pertain to vasopressors, inotropes, and antiarrhythmic drugs
2. List the various components that make up blood pressure
3. Compare and contrast the mechanism of action of inotropes and vasopressors
4. Describe the various drug interactions that may occur with the use of vasopressors and inotropes
5. Design an algorithm for the management of hypotension
6. Manage extravasation injuries that occur with use of vasopressor therapy
7. Describe the normal conduction of the heart
8. Define nonpharmacologic methods of treating dysrhythmias
9. Compare and contrast the categories of the Vaughan Williams classification system
10. Define the mechanism of action of digoxin
11. List all the dysrhythmias associated with cardiac arrest
12. Design an algorithm that may be used in the management of ventricular fibrillation and pulseless ventricular tachycardia
13. Design an algorithm that may be used in the management of torsades de pointes
14. Describe the proper dosage technique of intravenous magnesium therapy in the management of torsades de pointes
15. List the routes of administering medications during cardiac arrest

KEY TERMS AND DEFINITIONS

Match the following definitions with their terms.

1. _____ The presence of carbon dioxide aiding in the release and delivery of oxygen from hemoglobin.

2. _____ Amount of blood that is pumped out of the heart per unit of time.

3. _____ The lowest pressure reached right before ventricular ejection.

a. Antiarrhythmics
b. Atrioventricular (AV) node
c. Bohr effect
d. Cardiac output (CO)
e. Catecholamines
f. Diastolic blood pressure (DBP)
g. Mean arterial pressure (MAP)
h. Phosphodiesterase

4. _____ Pressure that drives blood into the tissues, averaged over the entire cardiac cycle.

5. _____ Cardiac medications that are classified according to their mechanism of action; in some instances, they may present multiple mechanisms of action.

6. _____ Endogenous products that are secreted into the bloodstream and travel to nerve endings to stimulate an excitatory response.

7. _____ Link between atrial depolarization and ventricular depolarization.

8. _____ Peak pressure reached during ventricular ejection.

9. _____ An episode of ventricular fibrillation, pulseless ventricular tachycardia, pulseless electrical activity, or asystole leading to loss of life.

10. _____ An enzyme responsible for the breakdown of cyclic adenosine 3′,5′-monophosphate (cAMP).

11. _____ Irregular heartbeat.

12. _____ An agent that influences the conduction of electrical impulses.

13. _____ An agent affecting the rate of contraction of the heart.

14. _____ A slow heart rate, typically defined as less than 60 beats/min.

15. _____ An overly rapid heartbeat, usually defined as greater than 100 beats/min in adults.

16. _____ A cardiac arrhythmia in which normal atrial contractions are replaced by rapid irregular twitchings of the muscular wall.

17. _____ A cardiac arrhythmia in which normal ventricular contractions are replaced by rapid movements of the ventricular muscle.

18. _____ Agent causing contraction of the capillaries and arteries.

19. _____ An agent affecting the strength of muscular contraction.

20. _____ An agent causing dilation of blood vessels.

i. Sudden cardiac death (SCD)
j. Systolic blood pressure (SBP)
k. Arrhythmia/dysrhythmia
l. Chronotropic
m. Tachycardia
n. Ventricular fibrillation
o. Inotropic
p. Vasodilator
q. Vasopressor
r. Atrial fibrillation
s. Bradycardia
t. Dromotropic

21. Tissue perfusion depends on what three factors?

    a. _____

    b. _____

    c. _____

22. If your patient was in cardiogenic shock and had a decreased cardiac output, would a pulse oximeter attached to his or her index finger be an accurate way to measure oxygenation status?

23. What is the major determinant of (a) blood pressure and (b) ventricular contractility?

    a. _____

    b. _____

24. Calculate the CO of a patient with a blood pressure of 120/70 mm Hg, a stroke volume of 70 mL/beat, and a heart rate of 80 beats/min.

25. What are two determinants of MAP?

    a. _____

    b. _____

26. Calculate the MAP of a patient who has a blood pressure of 120/90 mm Hg.

27. Define stroke volume.

List the normal pressures of each hemodynamic parameter.

28. Central venous pressure (CVP): _____

29. Pulmonary capillary wedge pressure (PCWP): _____

30. Cardiac output (CO): _____

31. Systemic vascular resistance (SVR): _____

AGENTS USED IN THE MANAGEMENT OF SHOCK

32. Your patient has just suffered severe blood loss due to the arterial line's becoming dislodged. What would be your first-line therapy to improve the hypotension?

33. Your patient's hemodynamic parameters are currently being measured. If the patient were fluid overloaded, what measurement would likely be altered? Would it increase or decrease?

34. List a clinical indication for the use of Levophed.

Catecholamines

35. After administration of epinephrine, stimulation of what receptor type is likely to produce a net effect of tachycardia?

36. Isoproterenol can be used to relax the smooth muscle of the bronchi. Why is its use limited? What is its brand name?

37. The medical student suggests the use of dopamine to treat a patient in septic shock. You suggest norepinephrine. How would you explain your choice and why it is the more appropriate pharmacologic treatment for the patient to the attending physician?

38. Explain why your patient receiving a phenylephrine infusion has developed reflex bradycardia.

39. Vasopressin (Pitressin) may be used for _____ shock.

40. Take a moment to go to the Surviving Sepsis website and check it out! http://www.survivingsepsis.org/Guidelines/Pages/default.aspx

41. List a clinical situation in which midodrine would be indicated.

42. List six clinical signs and symptoms of extravasation.

    a. _____

    b. _____

    c. _____

    d. _____

    e. _____

    f. _____

43. How can the risk of extravasation be minimized?

Inotropic Agents

44. List a clinical indication for dobutamine.

Phosphodiesterase Inhibitors

45. Why would you choose milrinone over inamrinone to manage your patient's hemodynamic status?

Cardiac Glycosides

46. Digoxin, the only drug in the cardiac glycoside class, is used in the management of chronic _____.

47. List four initial symptoms seen in digoxin toxicity.

a. _____

b. _____

c. _____

d. _____

ELECTROPHYSIOLOGY OF THE MYOCARDIUM

48. List the five major components of the heart's electrical conduction system.

a. _____

b. _____

c. _____

d. _____

e. _____

49. When is catheter ablation indicated? What is involved in the procedure? _____

PHARMACOLOGY OF ANTIARRHYTHMICS

50. Quinidine (Quinaglute) is used to treat atrial _____ and _____.

51. Procainamide is indicated in the treatment of _____ _____.

52. Lidocaine is used to control _____ arrhythmias, such as premature ventricular contraction (PVC), ventricular tachycardia, and ventricular fibrillation.

53. A patient with severe asthma is being treated in the cardiovascular intensive care unit (ICU) for hypertension with Lopressor. What is a potential side effect of this medication? Is there a better choice for your patient?

54. In general, amiodarone is used to treat _____ _____ arrhythmias.

55. Class IV drugs such as verapamil (Isoptin) and diltiazem (Cardizem) are referred to as _____-_____.

The following is a list of drugs used for advanced life support. Next to the drug give the indication for that drug.

56. Epinephrine: _____

57. Vasopressin: _____

58. Atropine: _____

59. Magnesium sulfate: _____

Answer the following questions.

60. When would intraosseous needle placement be indicated?

61. List the drugs that can be administered through an endotracheal tube (ETT) if IV access is not available.

   a. _____

   b. _____

   c. _____

   d. _____

   e. _____

NATIONAL BOARD OF RESPIRATORY CARE (NBRC) TESTING QUESTIONS

1. Pressure that drives blood into the tissues, averaged over the entire cardiac cycle, is:
   a. Systolic blood pressure
   b. Systemic vascular pressure
   c. Mean arterial pressure
   d. Diastolic blood pressure

2. A patient has a stroke volume of 70 mL/beat and a heart rate of 80 beats/min. What is the CO?
   a. 4.2 L/min
   b. 5.0 L/min
   c. 5.3 L/min
   d. 5.6 L/min

3. Which of the following pressures best evaluates a patient-specific response to fluid therapy and vasoactive therapy?
   a. CVP
   b. MAP
   c. Pulmonary artery pressure
   d. PCWP

4. The normal CO in an adult is:
   a. 8 to 10 L/min
   b. 5 to 7 L/min
   c. 1 to 3 L/min
   d. 10 to 12 L/min

5. Therapies used in the management of shock include:
   1. Fluids
   2. Inotropes
   3. Vasopressors
   4. Cardiac glycosides
      a. 1 and 2 only
      b. 1, 2, and 3 only
      c. 3 and 4 only
      d. 1, 2, 3, and 4

6. Norepinephrine and epinephrine are:
   a. Catecholamines
   b. Inotropes
   c. Calcium channel blockers
   d. Cardiac glycosides

7. Which of the following medications is best indicated for the management of septic shock?
   a. Dopamine (Inotropin)
   b. Vasopressin (Pitressin)
   c. Norepinephrine (Levophed)
   d. Digoxin (Lanoxin)

8. The only cardiac glycoside that is used in the management of chronic heart failure is:
   a. Dopamine
   b. Digoxin
   c. Dobutamine
   d. Epinephrine

9. Which of the following is *not* considered a major component of the heart's electrical conduction system?
   a. SA node
   b. AV node
   c. Bundle of His
   d. Mitral valve

10. Which of the following drugs is used for the treatment of life-threatening ventricular arrhythmias, such as ventricular tachycardia and torsades de pointes?
    a. Quinidine
    b. Procainamide
    c. Lidocaine
    d. Propranolol

11. Which of the following medications is a β-blocker?
    a. Metoprolol
    b. Vasopressin
    c. Magnesium sulfate
    d. Sodium bicarbonate

12. If IV access is not available in a patient with cardiac arrest, which of the following drugs can be administered through an ETT?
    1. Milrinone
    2. Epinephrine
    3. Atropine
    4. Naloxone
        a. 1 and 2 only
        b. 2 and 3 only
        c. 1, 2, and 4 only
        d. 2, 3, and 4 only

13. Which of the following statements is *false* regarding the administration of medications through the ETT of a patient in cardiac arrest?
    a. Medications should be placed in the ETT through a catheter that extends beyond the tip of the ETT.
    b. After medication insertion into the lung, 5 to 10 rapid ventilations with a handheld resuscitation bag should take place.
    c. Chest compressions should continue as drugs are administered through the ETT.
    d. Medications should be diluted with approximately 10 mL of normal saline when they are administered through the ETT.

14. Which of the following is defined as shock?
    a. A mean arterial pressure of less than 80 mm Hg
    b. Organ hypoperfusion and a decrease in oxygen delivery to tissues
    c. A CVP of less than 5 mm Hg and a Spo2 of less than 90%
    d. A reduction in heart rate less than 60 beats/min and a reduction in CVP less than 5 mm Hg

15. What is the MAP of a patient with a blood pressure of 110/80?
    a. 60 mm Hg
    b. 85 mm Hg
    c. 90 mm Hg
    d. 100 mm Hg

16. When administering medications down an ETT, how much normal saline should be used to dilute the medication?
    a. 5 mL
    b. 10 mL
    c. 12 mL
    d. 15 mL

17. SCD is defined as an episode of which of the following?
    1. Ventricular fibrillation
    2. Pulseless ventricular tachycardia
    3. Pulseless electrical activity
    4. Atrial fibrillation
        a. 1 and 2 only
        b. 2 and 3 only
        c. 1, 2, and 3 only
        d. 2, 3, and 4 only

18. What should be done *first* when a patient is in ventricular fibrillation?
    a. IV access
    b. Insertion of an oral airway
    c. Cardiopulmonary resuscitation (CPR) or defibrillation
    d. Insertion of an ETT

Chapter **21 Vasopressors, Inotropes, and Antiarrhythmic Agents**

19. Which of the following medications would be indicated to increase blood flow to the myocardium and the central nervous system during CPR?
    a. Epinephrine
    b. Atropine
    c. Sodium bicarbonate
    d. Magnesium sulfate

20. Which drug is most appropriate for patients, because of its chronotropic effects, in asystole and can be administered with epinephrine and vasopressin?
    a. Magnesium sulfate
    b. Sodium bicarbonate
    c. Atropine
    d. Vasopressin

CASE STUDY 1

A 19-year-old woman is brought into the emergency department (ED) by ambulance after an automobile crash. The paramedics tell you she has lost a lot of blood. She is intubated and being ventilated with a handheld resuscitation bag with 100% oxygen. She has IV access.

1. On the basis of this information, what shock state would you suspect?

2. Based on your answer to question 1, how would you expect the following hemodynamic parameters to be altered for this patient?

    a. Blood pressure: _____

    b. Heart rate: _____

    c. CVP: _____

    d. CO: _____

    e. SVR: _____

The patient begins to have multiple PVCs, and the doctor orders lidocaine. Her IV was inadvertently pulled out and currently no one has been able to reestablish access.

3. What could you recommend as a route of administration for the lidocaine?

IV access has been reestablished, and a CVP catheter has been inserted. The patient has been treated with various drugs and blood products, and her current hemodynamic parameters are as follows:
    Heart rate: 87 beats/min
    CVP: 9 mm Hg
    Blood pressure: 110/78 mm Hg

4. How would you interpret her hemodynamic status now?

An 82-year-old (53-kg) woman is in the ED by ambulance from a nursing home. During monitoring of the patient by electrocardiography (ECG) and while applying oxygen, the respiratory therapist recognizes the patient has gone into ventricular fibrillation. The patient becomes unconscious. Shaking and shouting have produced no response by the patient. The respiratory therapist initiates a CODE.

1. What is the first treatment that should be provided to the patient?

2. After this treatment, asystole appears on the ECG monitor. Which drugs would be indicated at this time?

3. What advanced airway could be provided to this patient other than an ETT?

4. After some time of performing CPR, the patient dies. In her chart, the cause of death is SCD. Besides ventricular fibrillation, what other dysrhythmias cause SCD?

Drugs Affecting Circulation: Antihypertensives, Antianginals, Antithrombotics

22

CHAPTER OUTLINE

Key Terms and Definitions
Hypertension
Hypertension Pharmacotherapy
Epidemiology, Etiology, and Pathophysiology of Angina
Antithrombotic Agents
National Board of Respiratory Care (NBRC) Testing Questions
Case Studies 1 and 2

CHAPTER OBJECTIVES

After answering the following questions, the reader should be able to:

1. Define terms that pertain to drugs affecting circulation: antihypertensives, antianginals, and antithrombotics
2. Categorize the stages of normal to high blood pressure
3. Define a hypertensive crisis, and differentiate between hypertensive emergency and hypertensive urgency
4. Design an algorithm for the pharmacotherapy of hypertension
5. Compare and contrast the clinical pharmacology of the agents used for hypertensive pharmacotherapy
6. Describe the chronotherapeutic effect of blood pressure, and design a pharmacotherapy regimen based on this principle
7. Describe the mechanism of action of angiotensin-converting enzyme inhibitors, calcium channel blockers, and β blockers
8. Compare and contrast the clinical pharmacology of spironolactone and eplerenone
9. List drug-drug interactions relevant to antihypertensives and plausible mechanisms
10. Describe the formation and elimination of an acute coronary thrombus
11. Describe the pathophysiology of angina and the drugs used to treat angina
12. List the agents in each of the following antithrombotic classes: anticoagulants, antiplatelets, and thrombolytics
13. Describe the mechanism of action of warfarin, direct oral anticoagulants (DOACs), heparin, and low-molecular-weight heparin (LMWH)
14. Compare and contrast the clinical pharmacology of heparin and LMWH
15. Describe clinical pharmacology of DOACs
16. List the laboratory parameters that may be used to monitor for the effect of heparin, LMWH, and direct thrombin inhibitors
17. Describe the mechanism of heparin-induced and warfarin-induced paradoxical thrombosis
18. Compare and contrast the clinical pharmacology of aspirin, clopidogrel, ticlopidine, and dipyridamole
19. Describe the role of genetic polymorphism in the antiplatelet activity of clopidogrel and anticoagulant effect of warfarin
20. Describe the indication and mechanism of action of glycoprotein IIb/IIIa inhibitors
21. List the indications and contraindication of thrombolytic agents

194

Copyright © 2024 by Elsevier Inc. All rights reserved.

Match the following definitions with their terms.

1. _____ Damage to the heart and the blood vessels or circulation, including the brain, kidney, and the eye.

2. _____ Maximal dose of a drug, beyond which it no longer exerts a therapeutic effect; however, its toxic effect increases.

3. _____ The volume of water filtered from the plasma by the kidney through the glomerular capillary walls into Bowman capsules per unit time.

4. _____ Neurotransmitter or hormone replacements that may be weaker or inert.

5. _____ Human biologic variations of rhythm within a 24-hour cycle.

6. _____ Treatment of disease by drug therapy.

7. _____ A drug influencing the contractility of a muscle (heart).

8. _____ Influencing the rate of rhythmic movements (the heartbeat).

9. _____ Drug that prevents or breaks up blood clots in conditions such as thrombosis or embolism.

10. _____ Measurement of the renal clearance of endogenous creatinine per unit time.

11. _____ Defined hemodynamically as the product of systemic vascular resistance and cardiac output (heart rate × stroke volume).

12. _____ Covalently cross-linked degradation fragments of the cross-linked fibrin polymer during plasmin-mediated fibrinolysis.

13. _____ Enzyme also known as *angiotensinogenase* that is released by the kidney in response to a lack of renal blood flow and is responsible for converting angiotensinogen into angiotensin I.

14 _____ Blood pressures higher than 180/120 mm Hg, with the elevation of blood pressure accompanied by acute, progressive target organ injury.

15. _____ Blood pressures higher than 180/120 mm Hg without signs or symptoms of acute target organ complications.

16. _____ Small peptides that result after the action of plasmin on fibrinogen and fibrin in the fibrinolytic process.

17. _____ Having the ability to activate and block adrenergic receptors; producing a net stimulatory effect on the sympathetic nervous system.

a. Antithrombotic
b. Arterial blood pressure
c. Cardiovascular disease (CVD)
d. Chronotropic
e. Circadian rhythm
f. Creatinine clearance
g. D-dimers
h. Dose-ceiling effect
i. Substitute neurotransmitters
j. Fibrinogen degradation products (FDPs)
k. Glomerular filtration rate (GFR)
l. Hypertensive emergency
m. Hypertensive urgency
n. Inotrope
o. Intrinsic sympathomimetic activity (ISA)
p. Pharmacotherapy
q. Renin

HYPERTENSION

18. List eight pathologies that may result from uncontrolled hypertension.

    a. _____

    b. _____

    c. _____

    d. _____

    e. _____

    f. _____

    g. _____

    h. _____

19. Clay is a 24-year-old Caucasian male with a history of insulin-dependent diabetes. His blood pressure over the past 6 months has gone from 138/82 mm Hg to 146/88 mm Hg. (a) Should he be treated pharmacologically for his blood pressure? (b) If so, what medication would you suggest?

    a. _____

    b. _____

20. How are blood pressure medications and doses adjusted?

21. Arterial blood pressure is a product of _____ and _____.

HYPERTENSION PHARMACOTHERAPY

22. How do angiotensin-converting enzyme (ACE) inhibitors work to lower blood pressure?

23. List two common side effects of ACE inhibitors.

    a. _____

    b. _____

24. How do angiotensin II receptor blockers (ARBs) work to lower blood pressure?

25. List a pathology that may require your patient to be prescribed a calcium channel blocker.

26. Describe the chronotropic effect exhibited by verapamil.

27. Fill in the table with the correct trade names of the generic calcium channel blockers available.

Generic Name	Trade Name
Verapamil	
Diltiazem	
Amlodipine	
Felodipine	
Nifedipine	

28. List six symptoms of β-blocker–induced pulmonary dysfunction.

    a. _____

    b. _____

    c. _____

    d. _____

    e. _____

    f. _____

29. Of the five classes of diuretics, which are most commonly used to manage hypertension?

    a. _____

    b. _____

30. List seven common side effects seen with thiazide and thiazide-like diuretics.

    a. _____

    b. _____

    c. _____

    d. _____

    e. _____

    f. _____

    g. _____

31. Your patient is a 31-year-old female with a history of hepatic cirrhosis. What medication would you suggest for treatment?

32. Glenda is a 62-year-old patient who has been taking eplerenone for many years as part of her heart failure and hypertension treatment regimen after her myocardial infarction (MI). She has recently been diagnosed with hyperkalemia and renal insufficiency. Should she be able to maintain her current regimen, or will the physician change her eplerenone to a different medication? Why or why not?

33. How do α_1 adrenergic receptor antagonists lower blood pressure?

Chapter **22** Drugs Affecting Circulation: Antihypertensives, Antianginals, Antithrombotics

EPIDEMIOLOGY, ETIOLOGY, AND PATHOPHYSIOLOGY OF ANGINA

34. List three symptoms exhibited by a patient experiencing angina.

    a. _____

    b. _____

    c. _____

35. How is angina pain relieved with nitrates such as nitroglycerin?

36. If a patient is at home experiencing angina pain, how should he or she take the nitroglycerin?

37. How often should nitroglycerin be administered for relief of angina pain?

38. What is the indication for ranolazine?

ANTITHROMBOTIC AGENTS

39. List three indications for heparin therapy.

    a. _____

    b. _____

    c. _____

40. Which has a longer time of onset, heparin or warfarin?

41. What is a concern when aspirin is given at high doses to patients with asthma and chronic obstructive pulmonary disease (COPD)?

42. List an indication of the use of Plavix.

43. List three indications for thrombolytic agents.

    a. _____

    b. _____

    c. _____

44. List two drawbacks seen with the use of warfarin.

    a. _____

    b. _____

45. Fill in the chart relating to new oral anticoagulants.

	Apixaban (Eliquis®)	Rivaroxaban (Xarelto®)	Dabigatran (Pradaxa®)
U.S. Food and Drug Administration (FDA) indication(s)			
Dosing			
Stroke prevention in nonvalvular atrial fibrillation			
Deep venous thrombosis (DVT)/pulmonary embolism (PE) treatment			
DVT/PE prophylaxis			
Cautions			
Contraindications			

46. List 10 absolute contraindications for thrombolytic treatment in acute stroke.

a. _____

b. _____

c. _____

d. _____

e. _____

f. _____

g. _____

h. _____

i. _____

j. _____

Chapter **22** Drugs Affecting Circulation: Antihypertensives, Antianginals, Antithrombotics

47. List two side effects of cilostazol.

a. _____

b. _____

NATIONAL BOARD OF RESPIRATORY CARE (NBRC) TESTING QUESTIONS

1. Which of the following is optimal blood pressure for adults 18 years of age or older?
   a. <120/<80 mm Hg
   b. >135/>85 mm Hg
   c. >140/>90 mm Hg
   d. <150/>70 mm Hg

2. Which of the statements is *true* regarding hypertension in adults?
   a. Hypertension is most commonly caused by smoking.
   b. The etiology of hypertension is unknown.
   c. Hypertension occurs less in the United States than other countries.
   d. Hypertension occurs more in nondiabetic patients.

3. Which of the following is the brand name for dabigatran?
   a. Coumadin
   b. Eliquis
   c. Xarelto
   d. Pradaxa

4. Which of the following are hemodynamic effects of ACE inhibitors?
   1. A reduction in peripheral arterial resistance
   2. An increase in cardiac output
   3. An increase in heart rate
   4. An increase in renal blood flow and unchanged GFR
      a. 1 and 2 only
      b. 3 and 4 only
      c. 1, 2, and 4 only
      d. 2, 3, and 4 only

5. What is the most common adverse effect associated with thrombolytic agents?
   a. Bleeding
   b. Clot formation
   c. Stroke
   d. MI

6. Most MIs, strokes, dysrhythmias, and venous thromboembolic events occur in the _____ _____, in concert with the circadian blood pressure peaks.
   a. Morning hours
   b. Afternoon hours
   c. Evening hours
   d. Relaxation hours

7. Which of the following pulmonary symptoms may occur with the administration of β blockers?
   1. Bronchospasm
   2. Wheezing
   3. Dyspnea
   4. Bleeding
      a. 1 and 2 only
      b. 2 and 3 only
      c. 2, 3, and 4 only
      d. 1, 2, and 3 only

8. Of the five classes of diuretics, which are most commonly used to manage hypertension?
   1. Thiazides
   2. Potassium-sparing agents
   3. Adrenergic agents
   4. Antiadrenergic agents
      a. 1 and 2 only
      b. 2 and 3 only
      c. 3 and 4 only
      d. 1 and 4 only

9. How do β_1 antagonists lower blood pressure?
   a. By affecting both cardiac output and glomerular filtration rate
   b. By increasing peripheral vascular resistance
   c. By blocking postsynaptic receptors
   d. By increasing the preload and afterload of the heart

10. Which of the following symptoms are exhibited by a patient experiencing angina?
    1. Chest tightness
    2. Pressure
    3. Burning sensation (indigestion)
    4. Pain radiating to left shoulder and jaw
       a. 1 and 2 only
       b. 2 and 3 only
       c. 1, 3, and 4 only
       d. 1, 2, 3, and 4

11. How is anginal pain relieved with nitrates such as nitroglycerin?
    a. Reduction in cardiac output
    b. Vasodilation of coronary arteries
    c. Peripheral vascular vasodilation
    d. Reduction in platelet adherence to peripheral vasculature

12. A patient with anginal pain was administered a nitroglycerin tablet 5 minutes ago. The patient has had no relief from the pain. What would you recommend?
    a. Seek emergency care.
    b. Wait 30 minutes before taking another nitroglycerin tablet.
    c. Take another nitroglycerin tablet immediately.
    d. Take two nitroglycerin tablets immediately.

13. Which of the following is an indication for heparin therapy?
    1. Prevention of venous thromboembolism
    2. Prevention of coronary artery vasoconstriction
    3. Prevention of platelet adhesion
    4. Prevention of pulmonary vascular vasoconstriction
       a. 1 only
       b. 4 only
       c. 2 and 3 only
       d. 2, 3, and 4 only

14. A patient has been prescribed warfarin. Indications for warfarin include:
    1. Venous thrombosis
    2. PE
    3. Congestive heart failure
    4. Mitral valve stenosis
       a. 1 and 2 only
       b. 3 and 4 only
       c. 1, 3, and 4 only
       d. 2, 3, and 4 only

Chapter **22** Drugs Affecting Circulation: Antihypertensives, Antianginals, Antithrombotics

15. What is a concern when aspirin is given at high doses to patients with asthma?
    a. It can induce severe bleeding from the gastrointestinal tract.
    b. It can exacerbate asthma symptoms.
    c. Minor bleeding may occur within the pulmonary tract.
    d. It can increase the changes of stroke.

16. Which of the following is a marker or symptom of myocardial ischemia?
    a. Angina
    b. Dizziness
    c. Tingling in the fingers
    d. Double vision

17. Sublingual nitroglycerin tablets lose potency after:
    a. 1 month
    b. 2 months
    c. 4 months
    d. 6 months

18. Which of the following laboratory tests is used to monitor the effects of heparin?
    a. Differential white blood cell count
    b. Activated partial thromboplastin time (aPTT)
    c. Bilirubin urea nitrogen (BUN)
    d. Extended bleed time (EBT)

19. Which of the following are antiplatelet agents?
    1. Enoxaparin (Lovenox)
    2. Warfarin sodium (Coumadin)
    3. Aspirin
    4. Clopidogrel (Plavix)
       a. 1 and 2 only
       b. 3 and 4 only
       c. 1, 3, and 4 only
       d. 1, 2, and 4 only

20. Primary or essential hypertension is the result of:
    a. Systolic blood pressure increasing 20 mm Hg per hour
    b. Diastolic blood pressure higher than 100 mm Hg
    c. High intake of salt
    d. An unknown cause

CASE STUDY 1

Mrs. A. is a 69-year-old woman with a history of hypertension and angina. She was treated in the hospital 4 months ago for angina with nitrates and an ACE inhibitor. She was sent home with nitroglycerin tablets and told to take one low-dose aspirin a day. This was the only episode of angina, and she has not had angina since then. Early one morning, Mrs. A. got out of bed and was washing her face. Suddenly, she began feeling light-headed with some mild chest discomfort. She turned to her husband and said: "I think I'm having another attack."

1. On the basis of her history, what do you think are Mrs. A.'s symptoms?

2. Mr. A. goes to the medicine cabinet to get nitroglycerin pills. He notices that the pills are 4 months old. Can he still use these pills?

3. Mrs. A. puts a nitroglycerin pill under her tongue. How long before she should start feeling relief?

4. It has been 5 minutes since taking the first nitroglycerin pill, and Mrs. A. has felt no relief from her symptoms. What would you recommend?

5. It has now been 15 minutes, and Mr. A. has given his wife three nitroglycerin pills. Mrs. A. has had no relief. What should Mr. A. do now?

CASE STUDY 2

You are a respiratory therapist working in the emergency department (ED) of a small, rural hospital. Because of the flu, the ED is short-staffed today, so you are assisting in other procedures to help out during this time. Currently, four patients are in the ED:
   Patient A is Mr. Wood, a 65-year-old black male.
   Patient B is Mrs. Gonzales, a 58-year-old white female.
   Patient C is Mr. Alexis, a 55-year-old white male.
   Patient D is Mrs. Allen, a 59-year-old black female.
   You are asked to take the blood pressure on each patient.

1. Which patient would most likely have hypertension?

After completing the blood pressure measurements on each patient, you record the following:
   Mr. Wood: 150/98 mm Hg
   Mrs. Gonzales: 120/90 mm Hg
   Mr. Alexis: 118/80 mm Hg
   Mrs. Allen: 132/86 mm Hg

2. Which patient would be considered to have hypertension?

On reading Mr. Wood's chart, you see a differential diagnosis of CVD.

3. Why would Mr. Wood have CVD?

4. If Mrs. Gonzales has a heart rate of 70 beats/min and stroke volume of 80 mL/beat of the heart, what would be her cardiac output?

After further evaluating Mr. Wood, the doctor has diagnosed him with uncomplicated hypertension.

5. What are first-line agents that can be used for uncomplicated hypertension?

After completing a physical examination on Mr. Alexis, you have found that he is taking warfarin. Mr. Alexis cannot remember how much of this drug he is taking and when the last time was that he took the drug.

6. What laboratory test can be ordered to determine the level of warfarin?

23 Sleep and Sleep Pharmacology

CHAPTER OUTLINE

Key Terms and Definitions
History of the Treatment of Sleep Disorders
Neurophysiologic Mechanisms
Sleep Disorders: Causes and Treatments
National Board for Respiratory Care (NBRC) Testing Questions
Case Studies 1 and 2

CHAPTER OBJECTIVES

After reading this chapter, the reader should be able to:

1. Define terms that pertain to sleep and sleep pharmacology
2. Describe sleep, its individual stages, and their electrophysiologic correlates
3. Comprehend the basic neurophysiologic mechanisms that promote brain arousal and wakefulness
4. Comprehend the basic neurophysiologic mechanisms that promote sleep onset and maintenance
5. Describe basic circadian processes and their interaction with the sleep-wake cycle
6. Recognize several sleep disorders that are amenable to pharmacotherapy
7. Describe the rationale for using certain classes of drugs to treat specific sleep-related disorders

KEY TERMS AND DEFINITIONS

Match the following definitions with their terms.

1. _____ Daytime sleepiness that is so great that it leads to inappropriate daytime napping or sleeping.

2. _____ A group of sleep disorders manifested by undesirable motor sensory or behavioral phenomena that occur during sleep.

3. _____ The approximately 24-hour cycle of biochemical, physiologic, and behavioral processes.

4. _____ Compounds that depress central nervous system activity.

5. _____ The measurement and recording of electroencephalography (EEG) activity, typically coupled with the measurement and recording of cardiorespiratory activity and eye movements, during sleep.

6. _____ The measurement and recording of the gross electrical activity of the brain.

7. _____ A class of drugs used to induce sleep.

8. _____ Drugs that reduce anxiety and promote muscle relaxation, and also promote sleep.

9. _____ Drugs that directly influence circadian mechanisms.

a. Parasomnia
b. Electroencephalography
c. Hypnotic
d. Barbiturates
e. Hypersomnia
f. Benzodiazepines
g. Circadian rhythm
h. Chronobiotics
i. Polysomnography

Answer or complete the following.

10. Until the mid-1960s, the field of sleep medicine focused primarily on describing and treating insomnia, parasomnias, which include _____ and _____, and hypersomnias, such as _____.

11. The respiratory therapist's role in sleep medicine is still evolving. During the course of a sleep study, what two roles does the respiratory therapist play when working with the physician?

   a._____

   b. _____

12. Approximately how many sleep disorders has The International Classification of Sleep Disorders Revised (ICSD-R) book has identified?

13. What may have been the first compound to be used as a sleep-inducing aid?

14. In the 1800s, Crawford Long, a surgeon in Georgia, employed the recreational drug _____ to induce sleep, amnesia, and pain relief for surgical procedures.

15. Give one reason why nonbenzodiazepine compounds and analogs of these compounds are used instead of benzodiazepine.

16. List three principal characteristics that the ideal hypnotic should possess.

   a. _____

   b. _____

   c. _____

17. List two medications that have been used in an effort to enhance ventilation in patients with high altitude–induced central sleep apnea or obesity-hypoventilation syndrome.

   a. _____

   b. _____

18. Somnambulation or _____ occurs during the first third of the night.

19. Several brain regions are involved in the active process of sleep, especially which two regions?

   a. _____

   b. _____

20. When determining the appropriate pharmaceutical intervention for a sleep disorder, what must be done first?

21. Normal human monophasic sleep has two stages. Name these two stages of sleep.

   a. _____

   b. _____

22. Nonrapid eye movement (NREM) can be categorized into what states of sleep (formerly known as stage 1 to stage 4)?

   a. _____

   b. _____

   c. _____

23. *Match the following concerning sleep stages.*

   1. _____ This stage was formally known as stage 1.

   2. _____ A person is in this sleep stage for 5% to 20% of the total sleep time (TST).

   3. _____ This sleep stage has EEG of relatively low voltage and 20% to 25% TST with lateral eye movements.

   4. _____ TST is 45% to 55%, with no eye movement and low chin muscle activity.

   5. _____ Electromyography (EMG) has high tonic activity, and the patient is in a relaxed wakefulness state.

   a. N1
   b. N2
   c. N3
   d. Awake
   e. Rapid eye movement (REM)

24. A normal sleep cycle begins with sleep stage _____ and proceeds through _____.

25. REM sleep usually first occurs within the first _____ minutes after sleep onset.

26. Adult humans typically sleep about _____ hours per night and spend almost one-third of their life sleeping.

NEUROPHYSIOLOGIC MECHANISMS

Answer or complete the following.

27. List two correlates that arose from observations seen in postmortem examinations of the brains of patients who died from *encephalitis lethargica* after World War I that relate to sleep.

   a. _____

   b. _____

28. Most ascending activation system (AAS) projections that mediate EEG arousal and wakefulness synapse in what brain region?

29. In general, how does sleep begin?

30. List the two components that influence sleep and sleep regulation.

   a. _____

   b. _____

31. Coffee and tea are used ubiquitously to increase alertness because these beverages contain _____, which is an adenosine receptor antagonist.

32. Circadian rhythms must depend on an internal _____ that is self-sustaining in the absence of external time cues and can be reset by changes in the environment.

33. Localized to the anterior hypothalamus, what brain region acts as the "biological clock" to coordinate the circadian rhythm?

34. Define *chronopharmacology* or *chronotherapeutics*.

35. Give two reasons why melatonin may be important to sleep regulation.

    a. _____

    b. _____

36. The hypnotic effect of melatonin depends on the _____ _____ of administration.

37. What medication approved by the U.S. Food and Drug Administration (FDA) for the treatment of the non–24-hour type of circadian rhythm sleep–wake disorder in totally blind patients?

SLEEP DISORDERS: CAUSES AND TREATMENTS

38. List five characteristics of insomnia.

    a. _____

    b. _____

    c. _____

    d. _____

    e. _____

39. A person with insomnia has some daytime complaints concerning the lack of sleep. Name four of these complaints.

    a. _____

    b. _____

    c. _____

    d. _____

40. The reduction in benzodiazepine use has coincided with the introduction of a structurally dissimilar group of _____ derivatives, such as the cyclopyrrolone agents.

41. Fill in the following table with the appropriate medication trade names.

Medication	Trade name
Estazolam	
Flurazepam	
Quazepam	
Temazepam	
Triazolam	
Eszopiclone	
Zaleplon	
Zolpidem	
Zolpidem CR	
Ramelteon	

42. A chronic and progressive neurologic disorder characterized by unpleasant sensations in the legs as well as a compelling urge to move them while the patient is awake is now recognized as _____ _____ _____.

43. What percentage of European and U.S. populations are affected with restless legs syndrome (RLS)?

44. Similar symptoms of the neurologic disorder in question 43 have incorrectly been identified as _____ in children.

45. This movement disorder is characterized by periodic episodes of spontaneous, repetitive, and highly stereotyped involuntary limb movements that occur during sleep.

46. List four diseases associated with late-onset RLS.

    a. _____

    b. _____

    c. _____

    d. _____

47. Multiple clinical trials have shown that dopamine-enhancing compounds such as _____ and _____ agonists were found to be the most effective for treatment of RLS and periodic limb movement disorder (PLMD).

48. When a patient is prescribed a dopaminergic medication for RLS symptom relief, what are some potential side effects?

49. In the original description of narcolepsy, persistent excessive daytime sleepiness and cataplexy (a sudden inability to move) were included. Name two additional features that have been also identified.

    a. _____

    b. _____

50. Name the three most frequently diagnosed primary sleep disorders in the United States.

    a. _____

    b. _____

    c. _____

51. Besides pharmacologic treatment of narcolepsy, other suggested nonpharmacologic treatments also exist. Name three nonpharmacologic treatments of narcolepsy.

    a. _____

    b. _____

    c. _____

52. _____ are undesirable motor, sensory, or behavioral phenomena that occur primarily during sleep. NREM parasomnia or arousal disorders include confusional arousals, sleep terrors, and sleep walking.

53. What three common factors do primary arousal disorders share?

   a. _____

   b. _____

   c. _____

54. True or False: Sleep terrors are similar to confusional arousals and occur during the first third of the night. Sleep terrors most frequently occur in children aged 5 to 7 years and appear with equal prevalence in boys and girls.

55. _____ or _____ occurs during NREM sleep and is characterized by the presence of automatic behaviors of varying complexity, including walking, eating, mumbling, and, rarely, violence.

56. True or False: The most common pharmaceutical treatment for REM and NREM sleep parasomnias is usually one of the longer-acting benzodiazepines.

57. True or False: A benzodiazepine taken in the evening to reduce the likelihood of experiencing an arousal event may induce residual sleepiness the next day.

NATIONAL BOARD FOR RESPIRATORY CARE (NBRC) TESTING QUESTIONS

1. A patient who is diagnosed with hypersomnia would be treated for:
   a. Sleep walking
   b. Night terror
   c. Narcolepsy
   d. Terror dreams

2. The first compound to induce sleep was the juice from the:
   a. Methadone plant
   b. Opium poppy
   c. Belladonna plant
   d. Eucalyptus plant

3. The modern era of anesthesia was ushered in with the use of:
   a. Ether
   b. Opium
   c. Cocaine
   d. Morphine

4. Although benzodiazepines are considered safe, side effects of these drugs include:
   1. Addiction
   2. Next-day sleepiness
   3. Incontinence
   4. Memory loss
      a. 1 and 2 only
      b. 2 and 4 only
      c. 1, 2, and 4 only
      d. 2, 3, and 4 only

5. A patient in the doctor's office is being prescribed a hypnotic. If you were the prescribing physician, what would you consider the "ideal" hypnotic to do?
    1. Induce rapid sleep
    2. Maintain sleep over 7 to 8 hours
    3. Have no residual effects on memory
    4. Allow minimal dreams during REM sleep state
        a. 1 and 2 only
        b. 2 and 4 only
        c. 1, 2, and 3 only
        d. 1, 2, and 4 only

6. Somnambulism occurs during which of the following sleep stages?
    a. N3
    b. N2
    c. N1
    d. Relaxed wakefulness

7. Which of the following neurotransmitters are involved in the production and maintenance of wakefulness?
    1. Histamine
    2. Norepinephrine
    3. Acetylcholine
    4. Anticholinesterase
        a. 1 and 3 only
        b. 2 and 4 only
        c. 1, 2, and 3 only
        d. 2, 3, and 4 only

8. When people awaken during this sleep state, dream recall is common. This sleep stage is:
    a. N1
    b. N2
    c. N3
    d. REM

9. This sleep stage has a patient exhibiting no eye movement and low chin muscle activity, and the person is in this sleep stage 45% to 55% of the total sleep time. This sleep stage is:
    a. N1
    b. N2
    c. N3
    d. REM

10. REM sleep usually occurs within _____ minutes after sleep onset.
    a. 90
    b. 30
    c. 15
    d. 60

11. Arousal and wakefulness are seen in a person by assessment of which of the following?
    a. Leg twitching
    b. Eye movement laterally and chin movement
    c. EEG
    d. Increased respiratory rate and heart rate

12. You have just pulled an "all nighter" preparing for your pharmacology examination on sleep disorders. You want to stay awake for this examination, so you decide to drink a beverage that is loaded with an adenosine receptor antagonist. Which of the following beverages would you drink?
    1. Coffee
    2. Tea
    3. Cola
    4. Milk (2%)
        a. 4 only
        b. 2 and 4 only
        c. 1, 2, and 3 only
        d. 2, 3, and 4 only

13. In addition to homeostatic need for sleep, sleepiness also depends on another major influence that relies on an internal pacemaker that is self-sustaining and can be reset by influence in the environment. This is referred to as the:
    a. Circadian rhythm
    b. Light/dark rhythm (L/D)
    c. 24-hour light/dark cycle (L/D)
    d. Daytime/nighttime cycle (D/N)

14. Which is a chronobiotic drug that is important for sleep regulation and has been shown to correlate with evening sleepiness?
    a. Levodopa
    b. Melatonin
    c. Dopamine
    d. Adenosine phosphate

15. A patient has come to the doctor's office with complaints of difficulty falling asleep, awakening frequently during the night, and inability to fall back to sleep. During the day, especially while driving, he falls asleep. This patient would have a diagnosis of:
    a. RLS
    b. Narcolepsy
    c. Obstructive sleep apnea
    d. Insomnia

16. A patient who is complaining of excessive daytime sleepiness and cataplexy would be diagnosed with:
    a. RLS
    b. Narcolepsy
    c. PLMD
    d. Insomnia

17. Which of the following is the most diagnosed primary sleep disorder in the United States?
    a. Narcolepsy
    b. RLS
    c. Sleep apnea
    d. Insomnia

18. The onset of narcoleptic symptoms typically occurs between what ages?
    a. 20 and 25 years of age
    b. 15 and 30 years of age
    c. 10 and 20 years of age
    d. 40 and 60 years of age

19. Conservative treatment of narcolepsy involves administration of which of the following medications?
    1. Stimulant for excessive daytime sleepiness
    2. Antidepressant for cataplexy
    3. Hypnotic for insomnia
    4. Hypnotic for fragmented nocturnal sleep
        a. 1 and 3 only
        b. 2 and 3 only
        c. 1, 2, and 4 only
        d. 1, 2, 3, and 4

20. Nonpharmacologic therapies that can be included in the overall treatment of narcolepsy are:
    1. Scheduled naps
    2. Regular sleep and awake schedules
    3. No eating after 6 pm
    4. Eight to 10 glasses of water daily
        a. 1 and 2 only
        b. 2 and 4 only
        c. 1, 2, and 3 only
        d. 2, 3, and 4 only

21. An undesirable motor, sensory, or behavioral phenomenon that occurs primarily during sleep is called:
    a. REM terror event
    b. NREM hallucination
    c. Parasomnia
    d. REM hallucination

22. A compound that depresses the central nervous system activity and has been used to treat epilepsy is called:
    a. Barbiturate
    b. Long-acting benzodiazepines
    c. Pergolide
    d. Cabergoline

23. NREM sleep parasomnias include which of the following arousals?
    1. Confusional arousals
    2. Sleep terrors
    3. Obstructive sleep apnea
    4. Somnambulation
        a. 1 and 3 only
        b. 1 and 4 only
        c. 1, 2, and 4 only
        d. 2, 3, and 4 only

24. Which of the following medications would you recommend for a patient diagnosed with RLS who also has had a medical history of hepatic disease?
    a. Pergolide
    b. Levodopa
    c. Ropinirole
    d. Cabergoline

25. Which of the following is the trade name of an immediate-release nonbenzodiazepine that is FDA approved for the treatment of insomnia?
    a. Ambien CR
    b. Rozerem
    c. Lunesta
    d. Restoril

Chapter **23 Sleep and Sleep Pharmacology**

Mrs. Polaski is in the doctor's office today for a physical examination. Mrs. Polaski is 65 years old, recently widowed, and retired within the past year from public school teaching. Her vital signs are normal, she is slightly overweight, and she has a very low activity level and performs no exercise other than walking her dog in the morning around the neighborhood. During her physical examination, she explains to the physician she feels she has insomnia. The physician asks: "What makes you think you have insomnia?"

1. What symptoms would Mrs. Polaski say she has for her to be diagnosed with insomnia?

2. What else in the patient's history would lead you to believe she has insomnia?

The doctor agrees that she probably has insomnia. Her physician decides to prescribe a 22-mg dose of temazepam (Restoril). She is instructed in the use of the drug and side effects and told to call the physician's office if she experiences any of these.

3. What are the side effects that should be discussed with Mrs. Polaski?

4. After some discussion about the side effects, Mrs. Polaski inquires about how she will know whether the drug is working and what should she expect concerning falling asleep and maintaining sleep throughout the night. What should she be told?

Two weeks after visiting her doctor, Mrs. Polaski calls the physician's office and wants to talk to the doctor about some of her issues with using this drug. She tells the nurse over the phone that since taking the drug prescribed to her, she feels like she is sleepier during the day and because of this has not even walked her dog in the evening. She also states that she seems to be having a greater loss of memory, which she did not have before taking the drug. For example, she puts things down, such as her glasses and cell phone, and cannot remember where she put them. She is also still awakening during the night, although not as much as before taking the drug.

5. What change in medication should be recommended?

6. What are some medications in both immediate-release and modified-release classes that could be prescribed to Mrs. Polaski? (Also include the trade name. You probably have seen these in commercials.)

CASE STUDY 2

Mr. Mart has come to the sleep clinic for an EEG to aid in a diagnosis of a possible sleep disorder. You are the respiratory therapist who will be performing the study. Observing the study is a respiratory therapy student from the local community college who is interested in entering the sleep medicine field. The patient has had the electrodes attached and continuous positive airway pressure (CPAP) mask fitted. The patient is currently in bed, with lights out, and the EEG has begun.

1. The student inquires: "It looks like the patient is not asleep but is relaxed. Is this a stage of sleep, and how do we know he is in this stage?"

2. Another question asked by the respiratory therapy student is: "Are distinct stages seen when a patient sleeps?"

3. The student then asks: "Is there a stage that a person remains in the longest in normal sleep?"

4. The inquisitive student then asks: "How will you know when the patient is in REM sleep?"

5. "OK," the student says, "So what distinguishes REM on the EEG?"